Much Madness, Divinest Sense

Women's Stories of Mental Health and Health Care

Edited by
Nili Kaplan-Myrth, MD, CCFP, PhD
Lori Hanson, MSC, PhD

Pottersfield Press, Lawrencetown Beach, Nova Scotia, Canada

Library and Archives Canada Cataloguing in Publication

Much madness, divinest sense : women's stories of mental health and health care / edited by Nili Kaplan-Myrth, MD, CCFP, PhD, Lori Hanson, MSc, PhD.
ISBN 978-1-988286-03-7 (softcover)
1. Women--Mental health. 2. Women--Medical care. I. Kaplan-Myrth, Nili, editor
II. Hanson, Lori, editor
RC451.4.W6M82 2017   616.890082   C2016-907371-8

Cover design: Gail LeBlanc

Pottersfield Press gratefully acknowledges the financial support of the Government of Canada through the Canada Book Fund for our publishing activities. We acknowledge the support of the Canada Council for the Arts. We are pleased to work in partnership with the Province of Nova Scotia to develop and promote our creative industries for the benefit of all Nova Scotians.

Pottersfield Press
83 Leslie Road
East Lawrencetown, Nova Scotia, Canada, B2Z 1P8
Website: www.PottersfieldPress.com
To order, phone 1-800-NIMBUS9 (1-800-646-2879) www.nimbus.ns.ca

Printed in Canada
Pottersfield Press is committed to preserving the environment and the appropriate harvesting of trees and has printed this book on Forest Stewardship Council ® certified paper.

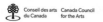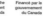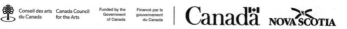

Much Madness is divinest Sense –
To a discerning Eye –
Much Sense – the starkest Madness –
'Tis the Majority
In this, as all, prevail –
Assent – and you are sane –
Demur – you're straightway dangerous –
And handled with a Chain –

– Emily Dickinson (circa 1862)

In loving memory of Tamara Ashley Levine, 1979-2016

Contents

For You,
As Validation of Your Struggles and Experiences

Nili Kaplan-Myrth and Lori Hanson

Several years ago, when we published *Women Who Care*, we seized an opportunity to share wonderful stories from women caregivers across Canada. The moment of inspiration was Dr. Kaplan-Myrth's distressed drive to Toronto to speak with an anthropologist friend about the lack of caring in health care. She returned to Ottawa and put out the call for submissions – her plea for others to share their experiences – and it was immediately off the ground. There was no uncertainty; we knew how to put together that initial collection and did so with verve.

Much Madness, Divinest Sense was also borne of Dr. Kaplan-Myrth's passion. As a feminist social scientist and a doctor, she was wary of medicine's history of pathologizing women. She questioned medicine's hierarchical framework, its construction and use of psychiatric diagnoses, and its abuses of psychopharmacology. Her research and her own patients' stories were rife with examples of misdiagnoses and approaches to care that cause significant harm. However, she also heard stories and witnessed ways in which medication and therapy very positively transform women's lives. What, she wondered, can we do to ensure emotional safety and empowerment in mental health care? How do women who are already vulnerable because of their mental health issues advocate for themselves in our health care system? Where are their voices?

Dr. Kaplan-Myrth also had a personal interest in mental health care. In her third year of medical school, she fell into a depression. She walked out of the role of caregiver and into the role of patient. She was cared for by a community psychiatrist who guided her through challenging years, taught her to trust interpersonal psychotherapy, encouraged her when she wavered in her personal and professional confidence. At her book launch, Dr. Kaplan-Myrth gave her psychiatrist an inscribed copy of *Women Who Care*. "Thank you for caring," she wrote.

Time passed and Dr. Kaplan-Myrth completed her medical training and family medicine residency. By the time she was in her second year of practice, she was faced daily with women patients who asked her to help them in their struggles with anxiety, depression, bipolar disorder, schizophrenia, eating disorders, obsessive-compulsive disorder, attention deficit, post-traumatic stress, chronic childhood trauma, and postpartum depression. They turned to her for supportive therapy. Her heart sank when she started to make referrals for psychiatric consults and received responses such as, "Sorry, we don't do trauma therapy at our psychiatric facility." She had patients with mental health issues who couldn't be seen by psychiatrists if they also had addiction issues. She had adolescent patients who wouldn't be accepted into youth mental health programs because they weren't in imminent danger of self-harm. She had patients with depression and autism who wouldn't be assessed by the psychiatric dual diagnosis team because they would only see people whose level of function was below the "bottom one per cent." When she asked for community psychiatrists who provided psychotherapy, she was told that their practices were full and advised that patients should access "other community resources." Subsidized therapy waiting lists were long, and private psychologists and social workers were financially out of reach to many of Dr. Kaplan-Myrth's patients.

It was time, she decided, to talk more honestly about the two-tiered mental health care system in Canada. It was also time to talk about how women are retraumatized by medicine's response to their psychiatric crises: women shut away in locked psychiatric wards; women stripped of their clothing and their dignity; medical staff's averted eyes and the lack of infrastructure for caring; psychiatry's ignorance or refusal to talk about trauma; mental health care providers who are too eager to medicate and sedate rather than to speak to women about their lives. And so she put out a call for submissions for *Much Madness, Divinest Sense: Women's Stories of Mental Health and Health Care*.

One of her co-editors, Dr. Hanson, was keen to be back on board. This was partly because of the positive outpouring of support for the first book and its powerful messages that readers repeatedly expressed "relating to." Also, like each of the contributors to this volume, Dr. Hanson had accumulated many life experiences with mental health, and questioned its verdicts and claims, recognizing its stigma and stories: a close friend and an aunt had both been hospitalized with severe depression; two young cousins lost to suicide; a second child recently (and disputably) diagnosed with bipolar disorder; decades of living with family members with addictions and trauma. Both editors were convinced this was a book that needed to be written. *Much Madness, Divinest Sense* was a new kind of risk; we were asking women across Canada to break the silence, to talk about the polluted, heart-wrenching, stigmatized, messy subject that is mental illness.

We who contributed to this book are putting ourselves out there: we ask you to contemplate our analyses of our experiences, to rethink the literature on women and mental health. We know that these are not the only stories that could be told about mental health; these are our stories. We also know that these are not the only versions of care; these are our experiences of care. Our goal is not to criticize individuals or institutions or models of care, but to spark discussion. We have deep respect for those who have dedicated their lives to caring for people with mental illnesses.

As editors, we risked putting together this collection of stories that are as raw as they are real. We made space for contradictory voices and opinions on the art and science of mental health. We suggest that nothing in this collection is sacrosanct. Our goal is to describe our experiences, as the recipients, providers, and critics of mental health care. Our hope is that this collection shines a ray of light on the dark halls and windowless rooms where historically women's mental health has been hidden from view.

I
Western Insanity and Women's Madness

We must try to return, in history, to that zero point in the course of madness at which madness is an undifferentiated experience ... This is doubtless an uncomfortable region. To explore it we must renounce the convenience of terminal truths, and never let ourselves be guided by what we may know of madness.

– Michel Foucault (1965)

A Brief History of Women and Mental Illness

Nili Kaplan-Myrth

What is Madness?

Madness, before it became mental illness, was deviance. "From the depths of the Middle Ages," according to Foucault, "a man was mad if his speech could not be said to form part of the common discourse of men" (1971: 216). In fourteenth-century Europe, it was believed there was a common thread shared among all people who rejected dominant beliefs, especially dominant religious beliefs. Included in this general category of mad person were heretics, magicians, sorcerers, midwives who delivered stillborn infants, alchemists, and astrologers.

In the sixteenth century, the burgeoning scientific enlightenment of the Renaissance led to, among other things, the emergence of the concept of the mind and then to the concept of mental illness. Although it was not until the nineteenth century that madness entered the domain of medicine, the effective discovery of the mind led to the popularization of madhouses. The opening in the seventeenth century of such institutions as l'Hôpital Général in Paris for the internment of mad people, criminals, beggars, vagabonds, prostitutes, the unemployed, and the poor led to this period being referred to as the "Great Confinement" (Foucault 1965).

Women in the seventeenth century were placed against their will in asylum wards reserved for deviant young women, prostitutes, unmarried pregnant women, and poor women (Chesler 1972). By the mid-eighteenth century, the strong influence of the Christian moral framework was reflected in the constitution of asylum wards: there was a clear ideological division between "virtuous" and "fallen" women (Weeks 1981). The general classification given to these inmates during the Classical period, from the mid-seventeenth to the mid-eighteenth century, was "unreasonable" rather than ill (Russell 1995).

In the nineteenth century, the rise of Evolutionism and the profound effect it had on the new system of taxonomy and the scientific method of classification led to the proclamation that "animality" was the essence of disease (Foucault 1965). This, in turn, led to the exculpation of responsibility for madness from the individual to the biological. The physician was then easily able to encompass madness within the domain of medicine. Nonetheless, the reconceptualization of madness as mental illness did not result in the total separation of the social from the biological. Instead, it empowered physicians to act as "moral guardians" in the prevention of the spread of the disease of "moral corruption" throughout society (Russell 1995).

It was far from coincidental that it was during the

nineteenth century that the "Woman Question" arose within the scientific discourse. Prior to the Industrial Revolution, women's participation in the domestic sphere had been considered of economic and political significance within society (Enrenreich & English 1978). However, scientists in the nineteenth century used the recent technological developments to secure men's place as economically and politically dominant while women were cast aside as dependent and inferior. Feminine quickly became synonymous with deficiency (Kirby 1994).

Given this scientific naturalization of women's subordination, women who deviated from their accepted position in society were considered "pathological" and treated accordingly (Matthews 1984). For instance, during this period, France used the following bases for committal in psychiatric institutions: those whose freedom was considered harmful to society; the young who disobeyed their parents and refused to work; single mothers; vagrant women; women of low intelligence; older people; women who led a debauched life, had loose morals, or were prone to vice; people who fantasized that they were someone else; and women who had consciously or unconsciously entered the sphere of politics (Russell 1995). It was at this point in the scientific discourse that the menstrual cycle, pregnancy, and menopause also came under the rubric of illness and deviance.

The incarceration of women by medicine did not relax as scientific research advanced. As Clarke insightfully remarks, "For the doctors, the myth of female frailty served two purposes. It helped disqualify women as healers but made women highly qualified as patients" (1983: 64). Elaine Showalter writes that "by the end of the [nineteenth] century, women had decisively taken the lead as psychiatric patients, a lead they have retained ever since, and in ever-increasing numbers" (in Russell 1995: 10).

The influence of Freud's discovery of the so-called "unconscious" in the late nineteenth century was to re-conceptualize the locus of woman's madness, moving it from her uterus to her mind (Enrenreich & English 1978: 126). A significant result of this transformation – in light of the dominant medical model of Cartesian duality in which the mind and body are considered separate domains – was a shift from concentration on invasive medical procedures such as hysterectomy to concentration on exploration of the mind through psychoanalysis. This meant that women's madness became thought of as psychogenic in origin, related to women's neuroses (Clarke 1983).

With the development and subsequent popularization of psychoanalytic theory, Freud used the unconscious and sexuality as the conceptual basis to reiterate woman's passivity and abnormality, and in so doing effectively perpetuated the medicalization and subordination of women. Although feminists such as Simone de Beauvoir relentlessly criticized the Freudian assumption that the female is a deviation from a male "norm" (Mitchell 1975: 308), the concept that it is "woman's normal state to be ill" continued to gain in social currency (Carroll & Niven 1993).

From the perspective of the early twenty-first century, it is clear there has been a dramatic transition not only in terms of the increased percentages of women undergoing psychiatric treatment, but also in respect to the increased number of women who have voluntarily sought psychiatric help.

Women's Untold Stories

Although there have been countless cases of women's madness throughout history, almost no personal accounts have been formally documented. Was there no one to listen to these women, to write down their thoughts? Is it an arbitrary oversight on the part of historiographers? Or perhaps these were intentional omissions, decided upon by historians, medical practitioners, and others with specific political agendas? In what contexts are women written into the history of human affairs, and when they have been included, in what sense is the writing critical?

Over the past few decades, feminist historians have laboured to demonstrate the academy's abysmal treatment of women: women are consistently excluded from historical accounts or, when they are not excluded, their subjectivity, self-representations, and experiences are denied, they are inserted obliquely as objects of the male gaze, and are situated in opposition to and almost always subordinate to male authority.

Accounts of the lives and experiences of "mad" women have suffered worse treatment than that of women in general by historians. To use Hardman's term (1973), mad women are essentially "muted groups." According to Astbury, members of these groups "become muted or are relatively less articulate compared with the dominant group because they have to express themselves through the structures and idioms of that group. It is not that muted groups can't speak but rather that they can't be heard" (1996: 26).

On the rare occasion that accounts of madness do emerge from the interstices of history, these must be approached critically. By and large, the only historical records of women's madness are in the form of psychiatric notes. In psychiatric accounts, women's madness is invariably reduced to symptomatological and aetiological factors, devoid of subjective or experiential elements. When confronted with mad women's protestations and self-representations, psychiatrists integrate these narratives into a biomedical framework.

"Posterity has treated the writings of mad people with enormous condescension," according to Porter. "Either they have been ignored altogether, or they have been treated just as cases" (1987: 2). Psychiatric myopia, so to speak, becomes a feature of historiography at the moment that psychiatric accounts are relied upon as a source of knowledge about women's madness. "Women," Astbury remarks, "are rendered most incomprehensible and muted by precisely those people whose professional credentials promise to provide them with their best chance of being well understood" (1996: 136).

How, then, can one escape the confines of psychiatric discourse and effectively enter into the realm of women's experiences of madness? It is possible to gain a better understanding of women's experiences than has been provided in psychiatric notes and in most historiographical accounts. To that end, I suggest we ask women to tell their own stories. The time has come to reinsert "mad" women's voices into our texts.

References

Astbury, Jill. (1996). *Crazy for You: The Making of Women's Madness*. Melbourne: Oxford University Press.

Carroll, Douglas and Catherine A. Niven. (1993). "Gender, Health and Stress." In D. Carroll & C.A. Niven (Eds.), *The*

Health Psychology of Women. (pp. 1-12). Camberwell: Australia.

Chesler, Phyllis. (1972). *Women and Madness.* New York: Avon.

Clarke, J.N. (1983). "Sexism, Feminism, and Medicalism: A Decade Review of Gender and Illness." *Sociology of Health and Illness.* 5(6), 62-82.

Enrenreich, Barbara and Deirdre English. (1978). *For Her Own Good: 150 Years of the Experts' Advice to Women.* New York: Anchor Press/Doubleday.

Foucault, Michel. (1965). *Madness and Civilization: A History of Insanity in the Age of Reason.* New York: Pantheon Books.

Foucault, Michel. (1971). *L'ordre du discours.* Paris: Gallimard.

Hardman, Charlotte. (1973). "Can There Be an Anthropology of Children?" *Journal of the Anthropological Society of Oxford 4,* 85-99.

Kirby, Vicki. (1994). "Viral Identities: Feminisms and Post Modernisms." In N. Grieve & A. Burns (Eds.) In *Australian Women: Contemporary Feminist Thought.* (pp. 121-133). Melbourne: Oxford University Press.

Matthews, Jill Julius. (1984). *Good and Mad Women: Mad Women in Twentieth-Century Australia.* Sydney: George Allen and Unwin.

Mitchell, Juliet. (1975). *Psychoanalysis and Feminism: Freud, Reich, Laing and Women.* New York: Vintage Books.

Porter, Roy. (1987). *A Social History of Madness: Stories of the Insane.* London: Weidenfeld and Nicolson.

Russell, Denise. (1995). *Women, Madness, and Medicine.* Cambridge, U.K.: Polity Press.

Weeks, Jeffrey. (1981). *Sex, Politics and Society: The Regulation of Sexuality Since 1800.* London: Longman.

II
Divinest Sense:
Our Stories

but if you look long enough,
eventually
you will be able to see me.
— Margaret Atwood
The Circle Game (1966)

Introduction:
Much Madness

Lori Hanson

The stories in this section insert themselves into history's sanitized record on women's madness with raw, angry, lonely, misunderstood, and hurting words. These are the voices of women[1] who have experienced mental illness as patients, as clients and as caregivers, as childhood trauma survivors, and as poverty-stricken mothers. Sometimes the experiences are like a roller coaster, with audible screams and visceral rushes; sometimes the voices barely whisper. Some women speak from secret dark places, and sometimes they have risen triumphant from a traumatic episode on the precipice of life. Some can scarcely afford the non-pharmacological treatment they want and need. In these stories there is more than a hint of the "divinest sense."

---

1. In some instances the authors used their real names and in others they adopted pseudonyms.

Bea Leaderman opens this chapter with *Escape in Sanity*. Bea immediately draws us in to the vulnerable place where her darkest moments are passing, full of fear and confusion; a place where she is, literally and figuratively, locked in. And the story unfolds.

In *The Garments of Secrecy*, Linda E. Clarke takes us below the surface of living with a mentally ill family member. Clarke's story is itself shrouded in allegory and metaphor, revealing secrecy to be ubiquitous in families loving and caring for someone who is mentally ill. "Secrets are eaten with the toast in the morning and the cold beans at suppertime … Secrecy is the caul of your birth."

Diane Reid begins her story in the darkest period of her life. Here we encounter the struggles of single parenting, poverty, and illness, a combination where "madness feeds upon itself." Support from her family, life in the countryside, and the love of caring friends lead finally to a bit of *Luck in the Darkness*, a transient luck, but "luck all the same."

In *Things We Put First*, Kay Tyler describes the many barriers that interfered with her ability to access care for her mental health. As a trans-identified woman, Kay was "afraid of being labelled crazy, afraid of medication … of not being able to transition." This meant Kay hid her depression from caregivers, even as she successfully became a woman.

Carol Casey's poem *The Escape* is a painful foray into the alienation and entrapment of "care," from which there is only one way out.

Mania "steals your soul and leaves you empty and alone." Kathy Evans' sometimes almost frantic prose reflects the constant state of alert that has been her lot in caring for her bipolar mother. A "parent" most of her life, the story is full of the raw emotion of a loving and dutiful daughter, keeping it all together, year after year. Only near the end of the story do we learn the true weight of care that Kathy carries.

Kathy's daughter, Shannon Evans, is wiser than her years. In *Caring in Advocacy,* Shannon tells another side of the family story, relaying a sister's confusing and painful journey. Rising above the personal struggles, Shannon advocates for her sister, and for all those who suffer from schizophrenia and other forms of mental illness. With her mother, she takes a vow and "we shift the conversation."

For Kayla Bathgate, the birth of her baby was not at all what she had expected. In *When Life Hands You Lemons: Postpartum Depression,* Kayla reveals the guilt at feeling disappointment after the birth of her child. Postpartum depression ends her dreams of breast-feeding, and eventually, though her husband is supportive, it threatens her marriage. But "gathering up the nerves," she encounters relief in a support group of mothers, and six months later, "it's hard to imagine" life without her baby boy.

Jayne Melville Whyte's story involves a long and tortuous search for the right diagnosis, and the right therapy. *Life Beyond Suicide* walks us through her almost fifty years in and out of the mental health system, forty of which she endured with a "daily desire to die." Ongoing struggles relay poverty, a system determined to medicate her, and ineffective therapies. She is now, however, "beyond endurance."

Misdiagnosis and a long search for the right therapy also feature in Kate Malachite's contribution. Spending eleven years on psychiatric drugs "to treat problems I didn't have" and experiencing agonizing drug withdrawal symptoms, Kate contends there is *No Quick Fix*.

It seems that the study of medicine produces its own mental health patients. In *It's Okay To Not Be Okay: Learning the Hard Way,* Kylie Riou shares her story of medical school-induced mental illness as a way to break the stigma of mental illness among medical students, in the hopes that they as physicians will become more compassionate and understanding.

In Sheila Morrison's story, *Caring for the Young Adult Child with Mental Illness,* a mother comes to the defense of her young daughter who is labelled a "behavioural problem" after her first episode of psychosis. It takes seven years before her daughter's diagnosis – micro-deletion 22q11.2 Syndrome or 22q – is identified and another eight years before her daughter is discharged home from institutions. Ever so carefully, with her fierce mother defender by her side, she begins to recover.

Esther Kohn-Bentley and Marty Hamer close the chapter with their touching stories, *Goodbye, Mamale* and *My Mother's Hands.* These are their reflections about how we age and the deep love between an aging mother and her daughter. Esther's Mamale is ninety-seven, frail, and suffering from mixed dementia. She is also a Holocaust survivor, a reality that a younger Esther embodied, living with vicarious PTSD, and "flashbacks and nightmares of events that weren't even ours." The question that has guided her life – "How can I make up for what they went through?" – seems answered by the precious moments she shares with her mother. Marty's descriptions of her mother's descent into dementia bring us from the first chaotic visit to an Emergency Department, to the long-term care admission, to her mother's bedside as she dies. Her mother's hand is the metaphor for industriousness, caring, continuity. "I took that hand in mine and I held on for dear life," she says. Even as their mothers' memories slip away, as they "lose their minds," Esther and Marty hold onto their mothers.

Escape in Sanity

Bea Leaderman

I

I hear the alarm keypad and the click of the door shutting above me. Most of the psychiatrists, on the first floor, left the building an hour ago. I could hear their voices, male and female. They said they'd check the bathroom, check Alice's office. I suppose they were looking for me. They didn't see me go downstairs. I am locked in.

I notice my breath, rapid and shallow, and I try to slow myself down. I am under a table, my knees cradled in my arms. I don't know how long I've been here.

Alice saw my tears and turned away, told me to pull myself together, told me to stop letting my emotions run the show. Maybe if she knew how scared I was, how sad, how fragile, she would come back to help me.

I have to pee. I look around me. I am in a carpeted room. There is a semi-circle of upholstered chairs, a coffee table, a wingback chair where she sits when she runs her group therapy sessions. A fake plant, a box of Kleenex.

There are two doors. I try the door adjacent to the table. It is locked. I crawl out of the room to try the door on the other side of the stairwell, also locked. I gaze up the stairs and consider: If I open the door at the top of the stairs, into the corridor, there is a toilet. There is also a chance that the alarm will go off.

I know the bathroom in the main corridor well. There was always a pink can of floral-scented spray next to the sink. And, across from the toilet, Picasso's Don Quixote, tilting at windmills.

I scamper back under the table and pull down my pants. I don't want to make a mess. I feel the relief as I start to pee into a box of Kleenex.

II

I am no longer thirty-nine. I am sixteen. In my friend's kitchen, I buckle over. I am not going to make it to her bathroom. I am too old to have an accident like this. My bladder is a metaphor as the world around me spirals into chaos. I consider climbing into their kitchen sink. No time. I grab a handful of paper towel and mop up the puddle, then head upstairs to a bedroom.

My legs chafe. Burning with shame.

III

I didn't have an accident two weeks earlier, the night my mother kicked me out of the house.

Slapped. Tears. I look down, my hair falls over my face. Door locks behind me. It is past midnight. I am on my own.

This isn't supposed to be my story.

It is November in Peterborough.

My breathing is shallow and fast, my glasses fog over. I can't see. My heart is racing. I am wearing a sweater over my shirt, jeans. The wool itches, makes me sneeze as I stumble down the block. The street lights are on, but the roads are pitch-black when I turn the corner.

I need a plan. I need to leave town.

I buy myself a Greyhound bus ticket to Toronto.

I need more from my house before I leave. My mother's changed the locks, so I shimmy through a basement window, a burglar in my own home.

I take my suitcase and dart to the bus depot. My ticket in hand, I wait.

What is my mother doing here? She grabs the suitcase out of my hands, dumps my clothing on the ground. The bus driver goes into the station, returns with a garbage bag, and offers it to me for my things.

I arrive in Toronto and I knock on my friend's door. Her parents invite me to live with them, no questions asked.

IV

I am in the basement of Alice's office, the stench of urine permeating the room.

I bear down and continue to pee. The Kleenex box overflows.

I send a text message: "I'm trapped." Alice doesn't respond. She gets the message but not the meaning.

My phone buzzes and my husband sends more texts. He asks where I am, if I am alright, when I will be home. He says Alice will be furious if she finds out I am in her office. She will phone the police if she finds me there, he warns. I am terrified. I write back to him again, "I'm trapped."

V

I stopped to pat my dog on my way out of my house that morning, then walked out the back door. I picked a few weeds from my front lawn and then headed toward my psychiatrist's office.

I walked on autopilot, roughly the same route I walked every week for five years. Alice was the woman I trusted with my story. Safety. If you crave it, you understand how important it is.

Alice greeted me in the waiting room each week with a smile. She ushered me down the hall and sat across from me, listening, as I gripped a pillow and alternately talked or wept. It was okay, she said, to be myself.

VI

I send the same message again: "I'm trapped." My friend writes back, "Where are you?" My mind is whirring. I can't tell her where I am. I know and I don't know.

Another text message arrives from my husband telling me that Alice is on her way. He's told her where I am.

I push a chair over to the wall, climb up to the window ledge, flip a latch, and the window slides open.

An alarm sounds. I am shimmying through a basement window again, into the dark night again, on my own again.

My black winter coat blankets me in shadow but doesn't keep out the wind. The sidewalks are treacherous, covered in thick ice.

I slow my pace as I walk past other people. They pay me no heed.

My phone rings a few minutes later, but I don't hear it. Alice leaves a message: "Were you trapped in my office? I am standing here and the window is open. You aren't here. I thought you meant you were trapped in your mind."

VII

I check into a hospital.

As I pad down the hall in stocking feet, the nurses refuse to make eye contact. I am not a person.

Nobody talks to me about childhood trauma. There are no social workers on the ward. There is no therapy of any kind. I decline sedatives and antipsychotics.

The hospital was a mistake. I get dressed and walk out the door of the ward. Nobody stops me.

I keep walking. Across town. Directly to Alice's office.

VIII

I ask the receptionist if I can speak to Alice and then I sit quietly in the waiting room.

I have a book to read. I wait.

I want to tell her how important she has been to

me, how helpful. I want to apologize for my tears.

Two hours pass. The last scheduled patient leaves her office. I stand up to ask the receptionist again if Alice will speak to me.

Police enter the waiting room. They confer with Alice and then turn to me.

"Alice, help me! Please talk to me!"

She turns her back and I am thrown on the ground. Handcuffs snap onto my wrists.

"Alice! Make them stop!"

I plead with the police to loosen the handcuffs. They push me out the door. I have stopped yelling. Sobbing, I ask them to be gentle with me.

When we reach the hospital, the psychiatric nurse tells me that I didn't have permission to leave, shouldn't have left. I thought I was there voluntarily. I did not know someone had decided I could not leave.

IX

Locked doors. Bare feet. Averted eyes. No offer of therapy.

Two weeks pass. My husband smuggles in my cell phone and I find a new psychiatrist for myself in the community.

I plan my departure.

Released.

Whatever it was that happened to me, it is over.

X

A year passes and it is winter again. I am out for dinner with my husband.

Alice enters the restaurant and sits down across from us, her back to me.

I wince.

I am strong, healthy.

I am torn: I want to yell at her. I want to hug her. The tug-of-war of attachment trauma: I ached for the mother I didn't have. Alice was the stand-in.

I understand. I mourn.

XI

And, now, here I am. I have my own clients whom I care for with empathy and compassion.

I am a good physician because I understand the complexities of people's lives. I understand trauma.

This is my story.

The Garments of Secrecy

Linda E. Clarke

Even though it's barely February, we opened the window a little last night to the air and the sound of rain and wind in the bare trees. The strange weather carried me in and out of sleep with ragged dreams of ships and getting caught below decks while the vessel heaved and tossed on the sea. I woke up time and again, hot and slick with sweat and with my heart pounding, pounding.

All night long, I tried to imagine how to tell a story that is a story about secrets. *My lips are sealed* came to me in the dark and rode with me the rest of the night. *Loose lips sink ships* floated to me as I woke up on the storm-tossed sea.

Secrets clothe the mentally ill and those who love them and care for them. Secrets paint the walls of the houses in which the families live, and secrets are eaten with the toast in the morning and the cold beans at suppertime. Secrets rode in the backseat of the car, especially in the dark when the windows were fogged by the breath of your friends. You were all grown up, although only a teenager, and they all laughed so easily and you stared out the window at the gritty snow and slush of the wintertime and tried to learn to laugh like they did. You did learn, in time, but only away from the secrets. You learned to laugh when you could leave the secrets behind.

You listen as this person tells the doctor that this person is just fine, thank you. And this person is fine, for the duration of the appointment. It has taken weeks and weeks to get to see this psychiatrist and you are gagged with anger and frustration. You want to holler: Remember the night you thought there were people coming to get you? Remember how you wanted to kill him the other night? Do you remember how you thought there were ribbons coming out of you?

The doctor tells this person how happy he is to see how well this person is doing. And then you drive this person back home. This person asks if you are angry or something and you choose to say nothing. You always choose to say nothing because it might rock the boat and everyone would sink.

To say one learns to wear the garments of secrecy is not really true. What is true is that you never knew anything else. Secrecy is the caul of your birth. You thought everyone lived this way, with grey in the house and the hollering and sadness and cold and the white-hot anger. It was only with the slow procession of time that you realized the secrets were not everyone's or everywhere. It was the slow procession of time that cleared your eyes, a little bit at first, and then a lot, of the red edges of pain.

But, still, your tongue is tied by the threads of the secrets.

And as you grow up and older, there is enough past behind you to know the truth. The garments of secrecy

don't fit anymore and you are awash in sadness and regret at the way the secrets shaped you and the lives of the
others who sailed that crazy ship with you. You didn't
have kids because of the threat of DNA and the remind-
ers of the ugliness of childhood. You didn't have a family because of the way the secrets were knives that cleaved
the space between you all. And that makes you shake
with anger — that the secrets of mental illness would
rather have you alone in the world than connected with
others. Secrets want nothing more than to be the centre
of attention forever and they will stop at nothing to quell
any light that might show them as they truly are. Secrets thrive in lies and the raw edges of cuts and the deep
bottles of pills and they thrive in time and time and time
again.

Can you imagine this? In the middle of one of those
nights she is called and the claw reaches out to her from
the hospital bed and the reedy voice scratches for more pills.
"Please, just one more pill." She says no. She offers comfort,
water. She says no again.

"You really are a cold-hearted bitch." The words are a
knife.

This past year has been a time of stripping of the
secrets and the lies that gird them and give them breath.
The stripping was a stripping of flesh, to the bone. Mental illness can do that to someone — bare them to the
bone. And leave them cold and without cover and without knives and without even pills. It can leave them pow-
erless and as needy as a newborn baby or maybe a dying
person who needs ice chips and company to help them
journey forward. No, not journey forward. Rather, to help
them be put back together again in a way that is a sem-
blance of the old self. Or, just maybe, help them be put

back together in the way they should have been years and lifetimes ago – your lifetime and theirs.

In the night, I heard a voice I remembered. In the heat of the summer, time turned languid and sleep fled. In the night, I heard repeated pleas for ease, repeated pleas for ease from the terror of the world at the doorstep. And there was nothing I could do but breathe and encourage and swallow my anger and fear, to smile and make tea and cook and lend a hand. Again. Always again.

We waited a long time, those of us who are tethered to this person, for the help that was needed, in spite of the way this person blocked it over and over again, in spite of the tower of lies that was built over many decades. All of that took pieces away from us. It took chunks of flesh and rivers of blood. Life will be shorter because of it.

Things seen cannot be unseen. Secrets do not work backwards. Once given air, they are dead and the truth appears on its old, numb legs. It has been bound up for so long. The sadness it carries can be as heavy as the world and the loss of the fantasy of the past can cut to the quick.

But that was a long time ago. Things now are okay. Now I am wanted, now I am loved. Now I am important. You tell yourself that over and over again, don't you? And you know it really isn't true.

But now you are grown up and you have the car keys and the eyesight and you have the wit to step in and help drive, advocate, fix, feed, pay, water, cook, laugh, try to bring joy. So you do it. But the clothing of secrets is put aside for only a bit. After all, there is no way to tell the story without baring peoples' bones to the air and that can bring pain because of the shame that all of this still carries. The shame is nothing new.

The garments of secrets are the emperor's new clothes. They are the garments of shame. They are as familiar to you as your own face, your own hand.

Luck in the Darkness

Diane Reid

I once went for three months without sleeping. No one believes me when I say this, understandably, but it's true. When I went without sleep for long periods of time, I found myself neither alive nor dead. For me, every moment was agony. When my mind wasn't busy trying to figure out the perfect way to kill myself, it raged with self-hatred.

Before the sleeplessness, I had been trying to earn enough money to support myself and my son. I was working hard at an overstimulating job. But then I was fired. My lack of income and my inability to pay off large debts, coupled with not qualifying for social assistance, sent me into a state of high anxiety. A few sleepless nights led to more anxiety, which eventually led to complete lack of sleep, and the beginning of the darkest period of my life.

Later, when I had passed through this black time,

I learned that one in five people are affected by what is variously called mood disorders, brain chemical imbalances, and madness. Regardless of the name, mental illness is a chameleon that manifests differently in different people and it can be hard to treat. So many factors are at play. Madness feeds upon itself. Lack of mental health makes it difficult to work. Lack of work leads to poverty, which leads to more mental instability. Many mentally ill become homeless; a large percentage of homeless people become mentally ill. I have lived in this tangled knot of circumstances, consequences, and illness. I hope by sharing some of what happened to me I can contribute to a dialogue that leads to better care for the mentally ill, in particular for women with or without children.

I was a young single mother when I became ill. Madness has a huge impact on family systems. It puts families off balance. In middle-class families, the relatively healthy partner has to take on all of the parenting while dealing with the grief of losing their spouse to an illness. The stigma around mental illness can keep the caregiver from seeking help. In a single-parent family the problems intensify. If the parent can't work due to her illness, the family income plummets. Poverty and madness lead to isolation and marginalization; marginalized people often lose their self-esteem as well as becoming angry and further depressed. Children become subject to inconsistent or non-existent care, and in some cases they are removed from their home.

In the '90s my home was small but safe. My son and I were building a good life, but it was a different life than I had imagined living. One day I needed cough syrup for him, and I did not have the money to buy it. I didn't have the money to enroll him in activities. I remember feeling like I lived a split existence: in my mind I believed I should raise my son as I had been raised, with all the benefits of a middle-class income, but I couldn't make this happen in reality. I was not in a position to work outside of the home, and when my mom found out about our circumstances, she began giving us money every month. It was the first – but definitely not the last – time she saved me from going lower than I could manage.

Time went by, and I began to feel like I could become financially self-sustaining. I took on a new job, and increased the number of fiddle students I was teaching. I was working hard, moving fast, feeling a little elevated in a way that I have since come to recognize precedes mania, and when I lost my job (no doubt due to the odd behaviours everyone but me could see), the shock increased my instability. I became more and more anxious, and eventually stopped sleeping.

To truly remember madness is to be mad, says Barbara Taylor in her book, *The Last Asylum* (2014). I can allow myself to remember only so much of what it felt like when I was severely ill. My son was seven years old when I had this first outbreak of madness. At the time I didn't know it, but I had mixed state manic depression, which involves racing, self-destructive thoughts. As the disease progressed, I began to think that I was infected by evil and that anyone who saw me would know this immediately. My fingers turned white; I thought I was becoming a phantom. I lay in bed, paralyzed, not going out, not wanting people to know my state of mind. When I did see people and they spoke to me, they sounded like they were coming from beyond the grave. A friend took me for a walk in the hopes it would help me feel better: I could see her skeleton. Many days I literally saw blackness: my vision was restricted to a hole in front of my face.

I don't want to complain. Many people have had it worse than me. I had a good house, I could borrow money to buy groceries and take my son on outings. I know that many ill people don't have that kind of financial support. I am describing my situation so that others may gain a little more understanding of mental illness and poverty, for even with help I was chronically poor. I also hope that other sufferers will find some resonance in my words.

When you are in a psychic place where no one else is, cannot earn your own money, and can't figure out what do with your child, self-hatred and shame set in. Looking back on that time, I'm not sure why I didn't ask for help from my son's grandmothers. My mind was so twisted and so detached from reality that I believed I couldn't ask for help. I hated myself for being a bad parent. My heart was breaking for my son, but I couldn't let him go. At the same time, in the broken pattern that is mental illness, I believed he would be better off without me. Even if he went to live with someone else I would still be a dark force in his life. To me, the only solution was to kill myself.

My son was most often with me, at home. He went to his father's on a regular basis, each time during which I would come close to committing suicide. When he was with me, I couldn't kill myself as I needed to care for him.

I have an active imagination. I can imagine what my life would have been like if I had not had financial help from my family. For certain I would have had to go to the food bank (later in my life I did use the food bank many times). I would have lost telephone service. I may have had to skip paying my rent, stay in emergency housing. I would have only been able to afford a one-bedroom apartment at the most. I would have been lucky to scrape up bus fare and might have had to walk everywhere. Walking because you do not have a car is not the same as walking for your health. Hauling groceries, taking children to appointments, trying to have a social life when it's forty below: these things wear on a person's soul.

If poverty had a colour it would be grey. Social assistance is simply not enough money to live on. You are forced to eat cheap food and feel hunger, which puts a strain on the mind. Good housing is hard to find and very expensive in Saskatoon; people on social assistance often live in cramped quarters. In the constant grind that is life on social assistance, it's easy to lose hope and it's hard to keep your temper. It's often been said that depression is anger turned inwards. Women on fixed incomes find themselves getting angry at their friends and families, becoming depressed, or both.

You have probably been wondering why I didn't seek medical help for my condition. I did go to my clinic, but my regular doctor had retired and none of the other doctors were taking new patients. I was allowed to see the duty doctor: she prescribed pills and didn't schedule a follow-up appointment. The pills did not help me sleep: in fact, they made me hallucinate. I was scared to continue taking medication without follow-up care, so I stopped.

At that time I was also seeking counselling. My clinic was able to put me on a waiting list, but the list was too long for me. I struck up a perfect plan to kill myself and one day I set out to the country with massive amounts of sleeping pills. I was looking for a quiet place to end my life. But I realized that no matter where I died someone would find my body and I didn't want to put anyone through such a gruesome experience. My plan wasn't perfect, after all. I turned for home and stopped by an old boyfriend's along the way. For the first time in months, I felt a glimmer of love and that glimmer was enough to keep me going through the long difficult years that followed.

That day I made a decision to keep living, but recovering from my illness was one of the most difficult things I have done in my life. The period during which I began counselling and later began medication continued to be as physically and emotionally agonizing as the early days of my bipolar disorder. Mental illnesses are not just in the mind; they are accompanied by painful physical symptoms: sometimes headaches resembling migraines, sometimes a painful crawling feeling all over the skin; sometimes both at once. When people are asked why they tried to kill themselves, they often say they just wanted relief from the pain.

Luckily, I eventually found medical help. My clinic offered free counselling, but only to people who had doctors at the clinic. They bent the rules for me. Finding a doctor was trickier. Then one day I remembered I had had a doctor at another clinic for my pregnancy and birth. I approached her, and again, luckily, she not only took me on but it turned out she often cared for people with mental illness living in poverty. She offered the kind of follow-up care I had wanted when I first started medication: she saw me once a week, then once every two weeks, then once a month as long as I felt I needed it.

Medication alone does not put madness into remission. You have to eat well, exercise, and search out the light wherever you can. Being alone intensifies the symptoms, but reaching out can be hard when you can't make sense of your surroundings.

Patience is a large part of keeping mental illness at bay. It takes time to get a diagnosis and time to accept it. It takes time to find the right medication and to find out what you need to stay healthy. The illness goes into remission, it comes back. Hope is key: my worst times were when I was hopeless.

Luck in the darkness is a funny kind of luck, but it is luck all the same. During the time I was at my worst I was only at peace when I was in the country, and many country-dwelling people stuck by me and offered help. One friend let me stay at her place whenever I was feeling particularly black. She would remind me that I didn't have to feel the way I was feeling. Another friend let me stay at her place for two weeks while my son stayed alternately with his dad and my mom, and while I tried to figure out where to live that would get me out of the city and cost less money than the place I was living in.

Poverty grinds hope out of people. My psychiatrist says she wishes she could prescribe financial stability. I have always tried my best to be financially self-sufficient, but usually you cannot work more than part-time when you are suffering from a mental illness. I have used the food bank. The workers and the clients are wonderful people. If someone gets a kind of food they don't like, or more of one particular item than they can use, they share. I told myself the food bank days were like Christmas. I never knew what I was going to get, and sometimes the food was incredibly good: organic milk, fresh greens, fruit juice. But much of the food was canned or processed. Over time my pride and my health began to slip and I hit a wall. One day I just couldn't go to the food bank any-more. I felt nauseous at the thought of food. Now, buying my own groceries is one of my favourite things to do. I buy healthy food and, when I run out, I eat brown rice. I feel wonderful. I didn't realize how rundown I had been getting while I was going to the food bank.

Most people in the western world don't find themselves alone, hungry and homeless, out of their minds, and worried about having their children taken away. But many do. And once a person is marginalized, the marginalization multiplies itself. Marginalization leads to disempowerment. I remember feeling like my circumstances were my fault. I needed a lawyer to help me get more child support, but I felt a lawyer would find me at fault as well. So I didn't get one. I felt like I didn't deserve friendship. I felt that former friends were too good for me, and I was in no shape to make new ones. Nonetheless, many friends stuck with me. I am very grateful for their ongoing support.

I have been up and down over the years, my medi-cations have had to be changed, I have often had to take time off work, and I have never been able to work full-time. I have run up debts. Now, my son has grown up and is living on his own. Having a child did not cause my breakdown, but worrying about having enough money to feed your child is difficult. Worrying about feeding your-self is less so.

When government child assistance programs ran out when my son turned eighteen, I had to figure out how to afford a place to live. I lived in a tent for six weeks the first fall after my son moved out. When the temperature started reaching minus ten at night, I turned to sleeping on a couch in my music studio. There was a washroom, but there was only enough hot water to fill a bucket so I took sponge baths. The waiting area had a kettle: I made instant soups. There was no fridge so I kept my food in my window. I lost weight. I felt on edge most of the time as I had to hide the fact that I was living in the studio. But I thought my bipolar disorder was firmly in remission, and I was working hard and talking to lots of people. Then one night I was taken to Saskatoon's mental health hospital in a police car.

The Dubé Centre is a beautiful new building on the edge of the Royal University Hospital in Saskatoon. It overlooks an even more beautiful river. The Centre is peaceful, the food is good, and the sheets are clean. I felt safe and cared for. I thought I knew what was real and what wasn't the night I went into the hospital. I was sure I was in a real life political spy thriller, trying to figure out who could be trusted and who couldn't. The doctors had to spike me with Ativan to stop my raving mind. When I woke up in the hospital and asked my friends what had happened, my memories were different from theirs. I had had a true break from reality.

I now realize that in the early 2000s, when I was hoping to kill myself, I also had had a true break from reality. I didn't want to go to the hospital. I didn't want my son to have the stigma of a mother who is hospitalized for mental illness. Besides, at that time Saskatoon had only a very tiny building to house in-patients and it was very difficult to get into that care. There are still not enough beds for psychiatric patients and there are certainly not enough preventative services to catch people before they free-fall over the brink.

I would like women to have the opportunity to have a family doctor. I would like these doctors to be familiar with the issues of poverty and mental illness. I would like to see programs providing part-time work for women with children and/or mental disabilities, and I would like mentally ill women to have home care and access to drop-in child care. I would like social assistance to keep up with the cost of living: fewer women would be under the intense stress that comes from not being able to make ends meet. I believe these steps would reduce mental illness and hospitalizations and save the health care system money.

Good care can put mental illness in remission. Most sufferers have episodes when they are not well followed by long stretches of time when they are fine as long as they take care of themselves. Much of the time I was in the hospital, my fellow patients were no different than my friends outside the grey stone walls.

Where would I have been if I had not been able to borrow money? I can't claim to know what it is like to lose my child to foster care due to a mental illness, or to lose my place to live because I can't pay my rent. My family's support has spared me, for the most part, from hunger and homelessness. I greatly respect women who have become completely marginalized. Each of them has her own story. I can't claim to speak for them. I can only write what I know.

References

Taylor, Barbara. (2014). *The Last Asylum: A Memoir of Madness.* Toronto: Penguin Hamish Hamilton.

Things We Put First

Kay Tyler

My name is Kay.

In 2007, my marriage of ten years was coming to an end, my self-esteem was non-existent, and I was depressed to the point of being suicidal. I was also facing the need to transition gender. My gender identity had been a problem I'd been avoiding for well over a decade at that point and it was clearly a problem that wasn't going away. If anything, it was getting louder and harder to ignore. I had a really good go at killing myself and then I made a friend who gave me some hope and a reason to keep going.

I started talking to a therapist with the hope of accessing a doctor who could prescribe hormone therapy. I didn't tell her how depressed I was. I didn't want roadblocks to transition. I was able to access HRT (hormone replacement therapy) and started living full-time as Kay in 2008, but I was still seriously depressed and still suicidal. I left notes for myself, reminding me that the blackness will pass and not to give in.

Years later, through that same friend, I found an amazing doctor who took me on as a patient. I don't recall how much I told her of what I was feeling. If I mentioned depression I'm certain I downplayed it. This doctor looked after my health and helped me access surgery for my transition.

Body-wise and life-wise I was Kay now. I felt like I fit in the world, but the depression still had me. It troubled my partner and caused me problems at work. In 2013, I started breaking down. One day, sitting in my truck in the parking lot of a hardware store, I realized that I just couldn't do it anymore. I called a crisis line and was able to speak to a nurse that afternoon.

Not many weeks later, I fell apart in my truck again. I hid under the dashboard and threw up. I couldn't make myself get out of the truck. My friend came and got me and took me to my doctor. My doctor, whom I hadn't trusted with my feelings, spent a great deal of time talking to me over the next few weeks. She found a medication that brought my depression to heel and she told me how to be kind to myself.

I'm stable now and the blackness is in check. How many years did I spend living with my depression because I was afraid to tell people – doctors and therapists? I was afraid of being labelled crazy. I was afraid of medication. I was afraid of not being able to transition. I was afraid that the people who could have helped me would have become barriers to my transition. So I kept my mouth shut.

The Escape

Carol Casey

She screamed into
their hollow ears,
wincing as the echo
struck her in the face.
And they watched her.

Her eyes filled with terror
and tears as she saw
behind their faces.
And they watched her closer.

She ran to the bars
of the cage, shaking and pounding,
calling for help.
And they drugged her.

While she was disarmed
they opened her up
and rummaged inside,

tossing among them
her delicate treasures
so that when she awoke
she wondered why
she could no longer walk
or dance, only crawl.

And then one day
she crawled away.

Mania

Kathy Evans

Mania steals your soul and leaves you empty and alone. I watched my mother experience this. The darkness of losing her son, then her daughter, then all her hard-earned and saved retirement funds. She moved into old age, living at poverty level with increasing mental and physical health care needs.

Growing up, I remember franticness. The storms that ravaged must have been dark and scary. They were to me and I felt like I was only on the edges of the tornado trying to weather the storm. Not inside like she was, unable to take control.

She wasn't always manic, though. A school friend who used to spend time in our home playing with me when we were thirteen years old calls from afar. She tells me she remembers I had "the best mother ever! Your mom made the best Jello and let us bake cakes!" I do remember a strong, confident woman who was a leader in her church. A lady involved in her community and local school. An active parent burning the trails, thinking outside the box, designing costumes and sewing them for the whole class for tap dancing, jazz, and baton recitals. There was nothing she was afraid of conquering. You want orange crowns for the pageant – crowns you shall have! She enlists my dad to bend coat hangers into multi-triangle shapes for a dozen crowns she will later cover with fabric and sequins. (I have kept mine – I feel magical like a princess when I think back to these younger years of my dancing!)

Such memories make it even sadder, seeing her now slowly slipping away, reduced to being childlike, needing help sorting out her medications, forgetting to put chicken boullion in soup, or needing help coordinating her plans for the day. Sometimes she doesn't feel like talking on the phone. She has given up her cell phone and computer as they are too confusing and stressful.

Over the years I watched a number of failed relationships that my mother pursued with men. She seemed to have the "seven-year itch," though my father did manage to stay with her for approximately twenty years. Through him I learned that my mother's behaviour had become chaotic in her older teen years. Incidents varied from ripping a phone out of the wall, to kicking her sister out of the house and throwing shoes at her in a burst of anger so she could not call the neighbours for help. There were many, but somehow Dad soldiered on. I learned as an adult that my father himself had been raised in a challenging home with his father admitted to the North Battlefield hospital (called the mental hospital then) when dad was a teen. So likely some of my mother's behaviour was somewhat "normal" to my dad.

I feel I have been a "parent" or "caregiver" most of my life, but I did have a few years of reprieve when my mother moved 1,200 miles away to care for her elderly mother. Distancing myself from my mother came at quite a cost to our relationship. She decided I was abusing my children and reported me to Social Services for spanking. Her behaviour was so out of control and unacceptable that I quit talking to her for a number of years. So she told her family I was a "horrible" daughter and that I had been the reason she moved.

Years later my mom was hospitalized. My uncle, her younger brother, called and asked me how long my mother had been ill. I replied, "My whole life." I had not known anything else. My uncle told me my mom wanted to apologize. They had put a restraining order on her and she could not go back to live with her mother, as she had physically assaulted her, pushing her into a brick fireplace. I did agree to talk to my mom on. the phone and she apologized. I then agreed to come and visit her. I learned that during that latest phase of her mania she had given away her life savings of over $100,000 in RRSPs to someone she had met on the internet. That news was shocking.

Over time, my mother was able to repair her relationship with her siblings. Being the oldest, she had promised my grandmother to never put her in a nursing home. She was allowed to move back into the home and care for her mother until her passing. My mother was fortunate to have had some estate money left for her care. The other siblings were given a lump sum while a trustee set up by her mother gave my mother a monthly allowance. She was very angry about this arrangement. However, the family knew she would need help with her finances or she would soon again be penniless.

When my grandmother passed away, I took time off to attend the funeral and assist my uncle and aunts in packing up the house and preparing my mother to move to her own apartment. Since my mother had also been a hoarder, this was quite the chore. The stress levels were high during this time, and my mother was full of anxiety. I spent most of my time gently working with her to prepare for the move and finding suitable accommodations. I had to return to work before the move took place.

She lived alone then for two or three years, but her health started to deteriorate. She started cutting her medications in half, speaking rapidly, and expressing incoherent thoughts. She began mixing up days and nights; driving miles away from home in the middle of the night and calling her sister saying she needed help and did not know where she was. She reported being "in a McDonald's somewhere." My aunt would get her to ask someone which McDonald's and upon finding out it was over a hundred miles away, she would go and bring her home.

The family realized the arrangement wasn't working. Finally, after three trips to the hospital in three days, she was admitted with dehydration and kidney failure. She was in trouble medically. Lithium and other medications which she had been on for fifty years had reduced her kidney function to one-third of normal. So they took her off medication. In her words, she "... felt she had just been handed her death sentence."

Her health continued to deteriorate both physically and mentally. More hospitalizations followed, including a three-week stay on the mental health ward. Her failing health required me to visit to assist with each emergency. Together with the crisis line, we were briefly able to put an intervention in place with mental health workers. But soon there was a downturn, and an emergency visit with hospital personnel advocating for her to be transferred to a mental health ward for appropriate care. This time, I visited again, experiencing not only the frustrations of the mental health care system but also the embarrassment of returning $1,200 of clothing bought over an eleven-hour period in the mania that had preceded the hospitalization. This was all part of caregiving that no one else was willing or able to do. It was exhausting. And after each trip I would retreat home and go back to work.

For me, this was the beginning of a journey on a new path in our relationship. Six months later, my mom is now on waiting lists for assisted living here in Canada. She has reconnected with her family doctor and psychiatrist. A kidney specialist has seen her, and her kidney function is improving. She has finally stopped losing weight and we have stabilized her diabetes with diet. Thankfully, no medication was required.

In terms of our relationship, it has been a long road to resettling. She originally planned to live with my adult daughter and myself. My daughter struggles with schizophrenia and bipolar disorder, which can make for interesting dynamics. My mother was to stay for a month while looking for her own housing. This has turned into a six-month stay. But through all of this, I am learning to enjoy the moments!

Caring in Advocacy

Shannon Evans

There are three responses to a psychotic episode, when sitting in a hospital waiting room. I see young nurses, terrified, staring. More experienced ones, averting their eyes, unseeing. Or what is possibly worse, pity. They pity my mother and me for sitting with our loved one, as though this experience were at all about us.

We are ushered into a room in Emergency, after hours of staring. The room is makeshift, more of a private waiting room than anything else. We're moved perhaps for our benefit, perhaps for the benefit of others. This is the stigma of mental health. I want to cry. I do. My sister curls up on the couch in her pajamas. You never get dressed in a crisis. She's exhausted from her inner battles. My mother, exhausted from caring for her. The continual care and advocacy for her daughter, this part of her that is hurting.

I go get coffee. Coffee won't help, but the walk to the hospital's Starbucks does. I can't breathe. I tell myself I should be able to stay longer, to have some endurance. I should be strong like my mother. Inexhaustible really. Yet hers is a story of a lifetime of mental illness.

My memories of our hospital trips are fragmented. I'm pursuing my education just metres away at the University of Saskatchewan campus, so I come and go from the hospital. I attend class, and try to breathe, but leave instead to cry in a stairwell. She is medicated now, her mind healing at the Dubé Centre for Mental Health. But her eyes are all I can think about. I see them when I close mine at night. Every facet of my sister has shifted. At this time, she's immersed in a medication fog, wherein even her laugh is not her own. Her humour is forced, her ambition stifled. Even with proper treatment, she's different than the sister I once knew.

Looking back, my sister's emergent mental health crisis blindsided me. I didn't know what schizoaffective meant, the first time. When we were young, all I knew was that my sister seemed obsessed with telling me far-fetched stories – conspiracies, almost. We grew up alongside each other with her experiencing mania, while I felt fearful. She became immersed in depression, and I, in overwhelming sadness.

All the while, I loved her. I just didn't understand. She would decide on a whim to run away. She claimed my parents had harmed her physically. I nearly believed her. I wondered if I had been the lucky one, kept safe for some reason. She would blast her music at different times. Loud music that sounded angry to me. My sister would change at a moment's notice. Wear vibrant colours, scarves, and hats. Having your sister accuse a youth

leader of being her father, her father of being a murderer
… watching her not engage in conversations, purposely,
spitefully – it was traumatic for me. Then, I saw my loved
one go catatonic. We had no diagnosis.

I have journals at the age of fourteen describing
what I felt: "I barely remember what happened last week,
or the week before. I feel numb, like I live through one
day and collapse into bed. Shouldering half of Mom's
burden … I don't understand what's going on with my
sister. I feel like she died inside. I miss the sister I used
to know." A month later, I wonder if she remembers what
she's said to me, mean things. I wonder if she remembers
me crying and looking her in the eyes. "Did she do it on
purpose?" I write. Two *years* later, she's manic. She tries
to bite my mom, take the car and drive, with wild eyes.
Mom takes the keys, my sister takes a swing; I take the
phone and call the police. We all wait, breathless. Can
you imagine? Not for my sister's protection, but for my
mom, for a record, for a diagnosis. I'm terrified, but good
things will come. First, another trial will come.

My most vivid memory of mania was her rambling,
non-stop, on the way to a barbeque. I can't shake it.
Mom, my sister, and I drove there – me, placating her in
conversation; Mom, driving the car, trying to make sense
of her words. Another moment – she sits in the school
gymnasium, eyes fluttering, rocking back and forth, and
clutching car keys again. Maybe she feels this might be an
escape. We convince her to get in the car. She sits in the
front, not replying to a word Mom says. When she did
speak, it was nonsense. "We've slain the dragon," she says,
with no emotion. I later write, "I hope she stays at the
hospital for a while. It's sad, but so true." I drop my mom
and sister off while they wait in Emergency. I drive across

the University Bridge, seventeen, and screaming until my throat is raw. I cry until I'm blind, and pull over.

They don't admit her that night. They didn't have a bed. She writes on colouring books and throws her shoes at walls, then Mom brings her home at two a.m. The following day, a miracle – she's admitted for two to three weeks. "Maybe we can get some rest now," I write. And we do, and we heal. Months go by. I miss my sister during this time, even though she's beside me. I deal with depression, lack of motivation and concentration. We grow; we're in a process of recovery. Mental health robbed us, but we go on. It's a process of oscillation. You take what you can, the pain, the memories. You cope. Then you grieve, and continue.

Why do I share this? I share to tell a story of caring. When someone you love is hurting, mentally or physically, you advocate for the best care. I understand that the behaviour and the person are not always one and the same. I will always persistently love my sister. I was young then but I learned from those first experiences. I learned to visit the next time she was hospitalized. I'm learning to tell her I love her, I support her, and I believe in her. I practise self-care, and see a counsellor. I'm pleased she does the same.

Sometimes to care is to advocate, to break stigmas, and raise awareness. One definition of advocacy describes a person who speaks or writes in support or defense of a person or cause; pleads for or on behalf of another. I vow to speak, to support, to strengthen another's message, to relate, and to grieve with. Sometimes to care is to paint with her, and go to movies. Despite being younger than her, I've always felt protective of my sister. I challenge people's thinking. I grieve when she grieves. I support her dreams. I partner with my mother to create lasting change, and help immediate family grasp the intricacies of mental health. We speak on behalf of a mental health organization; we shift the conversation. Here is our shared burden, and my story of being a young woman who cares.

When Life Hands You Lemons: Postpartum Depression

Kayla Bathgate

Postpartum depression. I'd heard of it and learned about it through our prenatal classes but never thought it was something I would be living with. I remember the night we learned about it in our prenatal classes and my husband asked me on the way home if I thought it was something we needed to be cautious of, given my history with depression. I said "no" and that "I was sure that part of my life was over and done with." Throughout my pregnancy, I felt so good and was so happy. Here I was, twenty-six years old, married to an amazing man, owned a home, had a loving dog and a baby on the way! Life could not get any better. I was already feeling such a connection and so much love for this little life growing inside of me that I thought there's no way I'm not going to be happy. At 6:26 a.m. on February 23, 2014, my world was turned upside down.

When our son was born, I didn't have the magical lovey-dovey feeling I always imagined. People had told me the feeling doesn't come for everyone, but that wasn't going to be me. I was going to fall head-over-heels in love with my baby the moment I saw him. Unfortunately, the feelings I actually had were completely opposite of that. At first, I thought I was just tired from not sleeping the night before and feeling overwhelmed, as any new mother would after just giving birth. These feelings would pass and we would carry on as a perfectly happy little family. But that did not happen and the feelings stayed.

At the time, I felt so guilty. I didn't want to harm myself or the baby – I just didn't want anything to do with him. He was supposed to come into our lives and give us warm, fuzzy, happy feelings. Instead, I felt completely empty inside. On top of the emotional disconnect I was having with my baby, I was struggling to nurse him. My husband and I had been gung-ho on breast-feeding and didn't see any other option. However, my emotional challenges along with some major latch issues put an end to our breast-feeding dreams really quickly. I sometimes think there were so many things I could have tried to make it work (i.e. a lactation consultant), but I was in such a poor place mentally that in hindsight, I don't think it would have made a difference.

For the first two weeks, my husband was the primary caregiver to our son. Once we switched to formula, I essentially didn't *have* to have anything to do with our baby. I would help out, but it felt like such a task. All I wanted to do was lie in bed and sleep. My husband encouraged me to take advantage of him being home for two weeks and get as much sleep as I could. I was so relieved that he was home but at the same time, as I lay in bed trying to sleep, I felt so guilty. I was this baby's mother and there I was lying in bed while my husband stayed up all night because the baby was hungry or had a tummy ache and wouldn't sleep. I felt completely hopeless knowing that after two weeks I was going to have to take care of this baby on my own, and I didn't have the slightest idea of how to do that. At the time, I didn't really care to try to learn how to do it, either. To be honest, I was regretting this whole decision. I wanted it to be a dream I could wake up from and everything would go back to being just me and my husband and our dog.

To make matters worse, as the days went on, my husband grew more angry and resentful towards me. I spoke to our midwives about how I was feeling and they said PPD typically wasn't diagnosed in the first two weeks because so many women suffer from the "baby blues." I kept telling my husband this, but he knew it was more than baby blues and was upset that I wasn't taking any steps to try to make myself feel better. He had battled through my depression with me before and was seeing the same traits reappear. He worried that he would go back to work and I wouldn't be able to cope on my own.

My mom had bought me *Down Came the Rain* by Brooke Shields. In it, Brooke pens her journey with PPD. I remember reading this book and absolutely bawling my eyes out. I was reading the same things I was feeling. On the one hand, it was reassuring I wasn't the only woman in the world who had felt this way but, on the other hand, it made me realize I was dealing with more than baby blues and that this was the beginning of a long, hard journey.

Finally, after feeling like my husband and I were

growing further and further apart and that I was not getting any better, I made the decision to contact my family doctor. He recommended I go on a low dosage antidepressant. I expressed my concern to him about anti-depressants if my feelings were in fact the baby blues. He said it would take the medication a few weeks to kick in so that if I started feeling better in the meantime, I could stop taking it. Meanwhile, our midwives had communicated with Families Matter and had asked them to get in contact with me to see if one of their programs might help.

Gathering up the nerve to attend my first group therapy session with Families Matter was hard. Not only was I afraid to leave the house with my baby (period!), but I was about to do so to express my feelings to a group of strangers. Luckily, within minutes of being there I knew this was the best decision I could have made for myself and for my family. To hear other women talk about the same emotions I was having was such a comfort. Comforting might seem terrible to say considering we were all there because we had PPD, but it was such a relief to be understood and not feel alone. My son and I have been attending weekly group therapy sessions for almost five months now and the steps we've taken are amazing. There are so many useful tools that Families Matter offers and being able to talk with moms dealing with the same struggles has been so helpful and inspiring in our recovery.

Now as I look at my son, who's almost six months old, playing away in his ExcerSaucer, it's difficult to imagine my life without him. I have grown to love him more than words could ever express and am finally start-ing to feel and experience what I always thought motherhood would be. Accepting PPD and asking for help was so hard, but I cannot imagine where we'd be if I hadn't done it. I don't generally like to use clichés, but I can say we're definitely within reach of that light at the end of the tunnel.

The biggest things I've learned throughout my journey are: Just because I have PPD doesn't mean I'm not a good mother. PPD does not mean I don't love my child. PPD exists and women need to know there are places and people out there that want to help. Don't be ashamed ... you didn't choose to have PPD.

My husband and I have always spoken very openly about our journey because we want to end the stigma that goes along with it (as with depression in general). We feel like the more mental health is talked about, the easier it might be for others to talk about it and ask for help. I would not wish the feelings I had on my worst enemy, but they are something I've accepted and grown from. I would encourage others having these same feelings to ask for help. You don't choose to have PPD, but you can choose how you deal with it.

Life Beyond Suicide

Jayne Melville Whyte

This is a personal reflection on the ten years of therapy since my last suicide attempt. The story contrasts the attitude of the formal psychiatric system for healing extreme trauma with the benefit of finding an experienced, flexible, and creative private therapist.

After almost fifty years in the mental health system, I am stronger and more confident and ready to tell my stories. My first twenty years of treatment frustrated me and the doctors. Then I was diagnosed in 1985 with Multiple Personality Disorder (MPD), now called Dissociative Identity Disorder (DID). I made progress through intensive work with the dissociative identity team in Winnipeg until it was disbanded. For a few years, the possibility of healing from the reality of childhood abuse was in fashion, but that belief didn't last. I moved back to Saskatchewan in 1992.

In 2004 I killed myself. I was fifty-six years old and

for forty years of that had endured a daily desire to die. When I regained consciousness, I was angry at God for sending me back, extending my life sentence. The psychiatrist asked me, "How could you do this to me?" With tubes in my throat, I did not have to answer.

To tell the truth, I hadn't done it to, for, or about him. Well, maybe a little. He could hospitalize me for safety but could not address or relieve the despair of my life. I refused more medications because I knew they didn't work. He called me a long-term stay who was spoiling his record of fast turn-around of hospital beds. And two days before the suicide, he had discharged me before he even took off his coat. In the previous seven years, this psychiatrist had never explored the MPD diagnosis in the literature or the trauma in my life. He hospitalized me when the community mental health workers became concerned about my safety. He charted "Depression" as my diagnosis.

When I returned from the intensive care unit to the psychiatric ward I'd left five days before, a parade of nurses and other staff visited to say they were glad I was alive. Several of them echoed the psychiatrist's question. I felt I was comforting them more than they reassured me.

For several years, two or three times a month I had been seeing a therapist, skilled in dealing with childhood trauma. Then the worker recommended a private psychologist. In my sessions with him, I went deeper into some of the memories, but he never allowed enough time at the end of a session to ground me back in present reality. I even took a timer that gave a fifteen-minute warning.

After my overdose, I was referred to the new psychologist in the public mental health clinic. She wondered, "If you've been in therapy for so many years, what could I teach you?" She explained she was not well prepared to deal with dissociated identities. We did not get beyond the second appointment.

One year after the attempt, I was hospitalized as a precaution. Before I accepted discharge, I found private counselling. With this resource, I have kept myself safe for the last ten years. The system saves money because I have minimal contact with the public clinic and no longer use the hospital. But therapy comes at a cost. I asked the health region to subsidize the fees, but they did not agree. Instead, I pay for therapy every month.

The practitioners generously subsidize me with a "volume discount." During a lifetime of mental illness, I was unable to sustain employment so my Canada Pension Plan is less than $200 per month and I have no private pension. With Old Age Security that began in January 2013, my pension is less than $1,000. At present, I earn enough from contract work to cover the two to four counsellor visits and a bodyworker session each month, $300 to $500. In addition, I am prescribed medication for diabetes, high blood pressure, and insomnia but also use a range of dietary supplements and complementary practitioners. There has been no communication between my family doctor and psychiatrist, and certainly none with my private health workers. So I am my own case manager; I have to be. Two years ago I sold my house and invested the money. At the rate I am drawing down my savings, I can afford to be healthy for another four or five years.

For the last three years, I have worked with a therapist who has previous experience with severe physical, emotional, and spiritual abuse. In the process, we began to untangle skeins of systematic programming and torture. She encourages honest and deep expression of feelings and creates a safe, loving space where I can learn to love and accept myself. During rough months, we make weekly appointments. If I leave a message, she will call back when she has a clear space. She doesn't phone in the few minutes between appointments because it is not fair to either of us if she has to rush away. I contract to look after myself and wait.

Routinely, I send my counsellor one or more emails reflecting on the previous session. Sometimes the emotions and thoughts that arise are not spoken in the therapeutic conversation. This may be especially true for clients with dissociation; I have commentators in my head while another part of me interacts. Often these observing parts write the notes to input their observations, fears, and realizations.

Between appointments, I email updates of my outside activities and my inside thoughts. Usually the therapist does not respond unless I specifically ask her to acknowledge receipt or to phone me. During crisis times, sending at least one email per day helps me feel more "in touch" not only with her but with myself. This non-intrusive communication also reassures her that I'm okay and will contact her if an attack of panic or despair threatens to overwhelm my coping.

Before each appointment, my email outlines the priorities that we (all parts of me) see and suggests a speakers' list based on who needs the most attention or has the most important issues. From time to time, we ask that she set out the foam mats before we enter the room as visual permission to pound, cry, and release the pain and horror of our memories. This freedom to make noise is a luxury because she works from her home instead of an office. Previous counsellors warned, "You could yell but there will be ten people at the door." Trauma often involved warnings about making noise and many therapeutic settings reinforce the silence.

Most therapists have insisted on physical distance. "You stay in your chair and I'll stay in mine," one said clearly. After asking permission each time, my current worker moves close enough to put her hand on my knee or take my hands. That touch makes it easier to maintain contact with her when I am drawn into trance states that transport me to former terror. Her calm voice reminds me to breathe, tells me I am safe, and invites me back to the reality of present time even as I explore the past. I can lie on her couch or rug when dealing with emotions that leave me no energy to stay upright.

At the beginning and end of each two-hour session, we share topics related to daily life. The closing conversation allows me to leave the intensity of the internal work and resume routine activities like grocery shopping or deciding to go home for a rest. After we confirm the next appointment time, she and I complete a series of grounding exercises, one of which requires moving legs and arms in a complex pattern that is impossible without being mindful. We stand up and walk around, looking out the window over her yard and garden, literally grounding in the sights of the changing seasons, before navigating the stairs to the main floor. By then I'm usually ready to drive.

When I spent time in the hospital, I often listened to patients whose stories suggested they would benefit from treatment for post-traumatic stress and dissociation, but psychiatrists were not making that kind of diagnosis, and instead were dulling misery with medication and erasing memory with shock treatments. Fortunately, my current psychiatrist has enough knowledge and experience to agree that medications are not the best practice for dissociation, but he seems skeptical about my diagnosis and my story. In my experience, there are not enough skilled therapists prepared to make the commitment for the complex and intense work needed to heal significant trauma. And cost is a significant barrier. I invest in my health each month, in time, energy, and money. I can't afford it, but I wouldn't live without it.

I've drafted a book based on the letters to my therapist written in 2013, telling my story and reflecting on the therapeutic and loving support that allowed me to find, feel, and heal my memories. Its title, *Beyond Endurance*, holds a double meaning. What I survived was beyond endurance. However, I've moved beyond mere endurance to live a full, useful, and meaningful life, as a writer, researcher, friend, and volunteer. I've made a commitment to stay alive and there are even some days when I don't need to kill myself. That's progress.

No Quick Fix:
A Story of DIY Recovery From Psychiatric Drugs and Misdiagnosis

Kate Malachite

(Adapted from the original, published October 7, 2013, by the Canadian Women's Health Network – www.cwhn.ca)

I am writing this piece because I have had terrible experiences with psychiatric drugs, and I hope some of what I learned while withdrawing from them may help people who are dealing with similar challenges.

I have been off psychiatric drugs since the spring of 2012, six months after I began withdrawing from them, and while things are not always easy, I feel much stronger and healthier. I hope my story can support people who are struggling. I am not suggesting anyone stop taking prescribed drugs. I can only speak to my experience. It took a long time, but I eventually figured out what was best for me. I wish that for everyone.

I was misdiagnosed and overprescribed drugs for years. And when I decided I wanted to stop taking them when I was thirty-four, I encountered huge resistance, was given terrible advice, and was left to sort things out on my own.

It is fair to say the experience almost killed me. There were a few times when I probably should have been hospitalized. I was mentally altered and actively suicidal. I was also desperate to stay out of the hospital because I knew I would be prescribed more drugs, and I would have trouble finding anyone who would believe that what I was experiencing was caused by withdrawal, not mental illness. I was lucky that I knew a couple of people who had seen withdrawal from psychiatric drugs before and were able to help me through it. They pointed me to the scant resources available on the topic, encouraged me not to give up, and, most importantly, affirmed that I wasn't losing my mind — I was experiencing rarely acknowledged but fairly typical psychiatric drug withdrawal, and I would eventually be okay. They broke the isolation I was feeling. I was also embarrassed that I had let this happen. I felt stupid for allowing myself to end up on a cocktail of psychiatric drugs that never really helped.

Over the past couple of years, I've realized this wasn't my fault. I was suffering. I wanted to feel better and my doctors wanted that for me, too. I became a living example of what can happen in a system that overprescribes psychiatric drugs, especially to women, because medication is generally perceived as the most accessible and least expensive form of treatment. Add to that rampant underestimation by health care professionals of how hard it is to get off these drugs and ignorance of the catastrophic withdrawal effects people often experience, and

I see that what happened to me is not at all unusual or surprising.

From age twenty-three to thirty-four, I was prescribed thirteen psychiatric drugs: eight antidepressants, three tranquilizers, a mood stabilizer, and an antipsychotic. There wasn't a time I was not medicated, and I never saw evidence that any of it was working. I was pretty sure the drugs weren't helping, but I was caught in a cycle of overprescribing and dependence I didn't fully understand until I started to withdraw from the drugs in the fall of 2011. It was then that I began educating myself about the issues because I was having terrible withdrawal symptoms and none of my health care providers seemed to know how to help.

I spent eleven years on psychiatric drugs to treat problems I didn't have. Over the years I was diagnosed with major depression, generalized anxiety disorder, and a few doctors even suggested I had bipolar disorder.

As it turned out, I was dealing with obsessive compulsive disorder (OCD). Living with undiagnosed and untreated OCD can cause unbearable stress in a person's life, and is usually accompanied by shame, stigma, and a sense that there is no way out. All of this can lead to depressive, isolating behaviours that superficially look like other mental health issues. OCD is far more complex than the pop culture image of a germaphobe who washes their hands too much or someone who checks repeatedly to make sure they locked the front door. It's not hard to diagnose if you know what to look for, but it seems that few mental health professionals are trained to probe for clues when part of the disorder itself is a compulsion to hide it out of misplaced guilt and shame.

Looking back, I see now that I started having OCD

symptoms when I was very young. I was seven years old when I realized I felt compelled to do things other people didn't think about. I remember asking a couple of grown-ups what I should do and they told me I was fine; I just needed to stop worrying about it. I suspected in my teens that I might have OCD when I saw something on television about it, but I didn't understand what it was – just that it seemed awful and I didn't want it. I hoped it would go away. None of the health care providers I saw over the years recognized my symptoms as OCD.

By my early thirties, it was clear to me that OCD was what I was dealing with and I couldn't avoid it anymore. The symptoms were so debilitating I could barely function. I had made progress with a psychodynamic psychotherapist on other issues, and I decided it was time to face OCD. I sought treatment at one of only a handful of specialized clinics in the country. Within a couple of months, I began seeing huge improvements. I felt like the puzzling mental health struggles I'd had my whole life were finally shifting because I had an accurate diagnosis and appropriate treatment.

At that point, I had been prescribed an improvised cocktail of an anti-psychotic (Seroquel), a mood stabilizer (Lithium), a benzodiazepine tranquilizer (Clonazepam), and an SSRI antidepressant (Zoloft). Every time I had a setback over the years, I was prescribed more drugs. The prescriptions were never meant to treat OCD, and, with the improvement in my symptoms, I decided it was time to stop taking medication I didn't need.

The doctor, nurse, and psychologist at my family clinic weren't very supportive of the idea. They didn't mind if I stopped taking Seroquel and Clonazepam, but they were reluctant to help me with Zoloft and Lithium, the drugs I had been on the longest. They stood by their various non-OCD diagnoses and thought I still needed drug treatment. I finally found a psychiatrist in October 2011 who set up a schedule for me to taper off the drugs.

I had been taking Zoloft for eight years. The psychiatrist prescribed half my usual dose for two weeks, and told me to then stop the drug completely. The drug taper seemed fast, but when I questioned him, he suggested I seek help elsewhere if that didn't sound right to me. With good reason, I didn't think I'd be able to find another doctor willing to help me. I followed his tapering schedule, against my better judgment.

By then, I had stopped taking Clonazepam. I had been taking it a few times a week for several years to treat anxiety attacks and to help me get to sleep. I was told to take it as needed and stop when I didn't need it anymore. I had noticed I had to take two or three pills to have the effect I'd had with one at first. I also noticed I was losing chunks of memory after I took them. I used to wake up in the morning and see that I had written comments on Facebook the night before that I absolutely did not remember. Since I was taking it only as needed, I figured I could stop any time. I learned later that taking a few benzodiazepines a month for several months would almost certainly create dependence. I had a prescription for thirty pills a month on an annual repeat. I never took that many, but I took enough to have unknowingly become dependent on them.

I had also gradually come off the anti-psychotic, which I had started a few months earlier when I was having severe PMS symptoms. The team at the family clinic suggested that Seroquel, a potent anti-psychotic used to treat schizophrenia and bipolar disorder, had been shown when taken at a much lower dose to help PMS symptoms. I was wary, but as had often been the case when psychiatric drugs were prescribed, the implication was that if I really wanted to help myself, I'd give their suggestion a try. Even at one-eighth the recommended dose, I felt like a zombie. I slurred my speech, slept twelve to fourteen hours a day, and had trouble concentrating. I hated it. I felt lethargic and light-headed during the tapering, but better as soon as the drug was out of my system. The most severe symptoms I had were electric zap-like sensations in my brain, drooling, relentless motion sickness, slurred speech, sweats, memory and coordination problems, restless legs, and tremors. I called the psychiatrist and my family clinic and both insisted I was having a relapse. I knew I wasn't, but couldn't find anyone who believed me and could help. This is the point, from what I have heard from dozens of people over the past year, when most people give up and go back on the drug. Their withdrawal symptoms go away, but they are still on a drug they want to stop taking.

The message here isn't that people should avoid psychiatric drugs. Some people do very well with them, and that cannot be discounted. From what I have seen, the problem is when diagnoses are made hastily, medications are prescribed freely, and there is a dangerous lack of understanding about the long-term consequences of these practices in people's lives. Compound that with the prevailing refusal within the biomedical system to listen to people once they have a mental illness diagnosis or are taking psychiatric medication, and it's a real mess.

Many of us might benefit from psychotherapy more than psychopharmacology. That has certainly been my experience. It works really well, but it isn't easy. Therapy with a clinical psychologist is expensive and doesn't claim to provide the instant relief that pills supposedly do. And it's not covered by provincial health plans. Psychiatric care is covered, but in an overwhelmed system, most psychiatrists don't offer therapy – they provide diagnoses and recommend medications.

The way our health care system is structured, pills are generally perceived as cheaper and simpler than psychotherapy because many prescriptions are covered by provincial health insurance plans while psychotherapy has limited or no insurance coverage. Many people who are having mental health issues can't afford psychotherapy. But lots of people can afford medication. Other potentially helpful non-drug treatments, like acupuncture and biofeedback, are also financially out of reach for many people because they are costly and rarely covered by insurance.

This speaks to the pharmaceutical industry's influence on what treatments public and private health insurance plans will cover and, consequently, the way people are treated for psychiatric conditions. The system is set up to prioritize drug interventions, and that can lead to devastating consequences for people who would do better with other therapies.

In an ideal world, diagnoses would be made based on attentive, compassionate assessments, psychotherapy would be available to anyone who wanted it, and psychiatric drugs would not be the default treatment when people are struggling emotionally.

It's Okay To Not Be Okay:
Learning the Hard Way

Kylie Riou

Never before medical school have I talked so much about wellness, how to prevent disease, and how to take care of patients, without any thought of what this meant for myself in my own life. I have shared my story a few times, with a few different medical student cohorts. The reason I keep sharing and shedding light on my own mental illness journey is twofold. Firstly, because it holds me accountable to my own wellness – maintaining my resilience and practising what I preach – and secondly, because I don't think my experiences with anxiety, depression, and burnout are unique. A large part of me believes that I experienced what I did in order to share it, to talk about it, and to help bring about positive and lasting change.

In no way am I an expert on wellness, an expert on medical education, or an expert on mental health. I will consider my contribution worthwhile if it empowers even a single person to seek help, to share his/her story, or to join me in stopping the stigma around mental health.

As a medical professional, I review many academic journals and articles in my day-to-day life. Evidence in the literature is absolutely overwhelming about stress, burnout, and mental health issues in every population. Specifically, it is also overwhelming where it pertains to medical students, residents, and our physicians. What isn't overwhelming is people talking about it, sharing their stories, and joining the discussion on figuring out how to prevent, predict, and properly address wellness and mental health issues.

When I was twenty years old I entered medical school. I started out as a spry young grasshopper. I had completed two years of undergraduate training and was so nervous about starting medical school. I had a steep learning curve, a brand new cohort of peers, and a desire to bring about change. I learned anatomy and physiology, tried to love histology (the study of disease at the cellular level), and made friends with other physicians, calling them by their first name. I probably partied a little too hard, but I did well academically, and practised percussing all of the walls in my house. Around April of my first year, I got bitten by the "need to make a difference" bug, and applied to be the Student Medical Society of Saskatchewan president. This was roughly a thirty-to-forty-hour per week commitment on top of a very busy schedule. In addition to the regular curriculum, plus my leadership role, I was also involved in an extra Global Health curriculum called "Making the Links," which involved two extra courses, spending summers in northern Saskatchewan and rural Nicaragua, and volunteering at the student-run clinic SWITCH in the inner city of Saskatoon.

Once second year started I hit the ground running … and running … and running. Between my commitments of presidency, the regular curriculum, and Making the Links, my schedule left little time for anything else. My relationships with friends and family, my healthy eating and exercise habits, and my study time all suffered. However, in the midst of all of these very large commitments, I kept waiting for the stress, anxiety, and worry to pass – and for the most part, it did. I had time to rest, to rejuvenate, and to try to be "well."

Then third year of medical school came around, and while it wasn't relaxed, it was much more manageable. I fulfilled my commitments for the Global Health course, finally had time to give the focus and attention to my studies that they needed, and catch up with old friends, family, and enjoyable activities I had been neglecting. The thing was, I couldn't get out of bed to make it to a single obstetrics and gynecology lecture. I was tired, I was burnt-out, and I was unmotivated. Although during my presidency I had found joy in sending fifty to a hundred emails a day, now I had no joy. I had been a classic medical student overachiever, and organized, efficient, and productive were my middle names. This all became rather muddled in my third year.

I wasn't happy hanging out with friends, and increasingly I became isolated, and felt extremely overwhelmed, despite the significant decrease in commitments. Nevertheless, I muddled along, finished the first half of my third year, and managed to pass all the comprehensive exams. I had three weeks off at Christmas. I spent time with my family and friends and felt refreshed.

Yet I was terrified for what was coming in third and fourth year – my clinical clerkship (JURSI: Junior Under-graduate Rotating Student Internship).

I started this new chapter on Internal Medicine and completed a rotation in gastroenterology, neurology, and infectious disease. These six weeks passed by without the events I convinced myself would happen – such as embarrassment, mistakes that would hurt patients, and never knowing enough. After that I was onto my elective rotations, travelling to Calgary, Edmonton, and throughout Saskatoon to complete these. Again, thankfully, all went well. But given my desire to impress my preceptors, each came with a significant amount of stress, and in my downtime I was irritable, unhappy, and not myself as friends, roommates, and my partner at the time could attest to.

Increasingly, I found it difficult to study. I began sleeping all the time and was disinterested in what I used to be passionate about. I felt guilty toward all of the people I was letting down. I had little to no energy, couldn't concentrate to save my life, had no appetite, and had become stiff and slow and sad. I basically went through a common depression screening tool in my mind over and over, and I lit up like a Christmas tree. I was a walking ball of stress, anxiety, and depression.

Like many medical professionals, I am a Type A person, and I told myself, "I will get past this. I can't let anyone know." How could I admit weakness? My struggles felt like absolute failure.

The situation went from bad to worse. Life began to look like a bleak, rainy, November day. I had stopped exercising altogether, I was eating way too much unhealthy food, and every time I sat down to study my eyes would fill with tears and my stomach would become a knot of anxiety. I was so overwhelmed at how stupid and inadequate I felt that I couldn't fathom studying because I knew I was hopeless. I started a new rotation, on anesthesia, and I started to have panic attacks before my shifts. I was so anxious about starting an intravenous line or intubating a patient and failing. I was so scared to be judged as inadequate that it contributed to a poor performance.

Throughout those dark months I completely shut out the ones who loved me most. I stopped calling and answering my parents' phone calls, I made up excuses to friends so as not to see them, I avoided my roommates, and I bailed on academic commitments. I believe many people noticed a change, but another thing common to the medical profession is that of empathizing with another person's struggles, and then normalizing what is not normal behaviour or coping mechanisms.

The most prominent emotion and feeling for me throughout all of this was the feeling of utter and complete isolation. I felt like everyone else in my cohort of medical students was successfully completing their rotations, loving life, and excelling in whatever they put their minds to. I felt like I was the only one having a difficult time, and that nobody else could begin to relate.

I was questioning why I was even in medicine on a daily basis. At this point I couldn't study, I was convinced I was going to fail out of medical school, and I constantly berated myself, internally reiterating that I was a pathetic loser who couldn't get out of bed.

Over and over again, these thoughts would cycle through my head, making me sick to my stomach. I felt like my life had no meaning. I was as far away from my faith as I had ever been, and was avoiding my church community like the plague.

Martha Manning has a particularly powerful quote that I believe aptly describes how I felt during all of this: "Depression is such a cruel punishment. There are no fevers, no rashes, no blood tests to send people scurrying in concern, just the slow erosion of self, as insidious as cancer. And, like cancer, it is essentially a solitary experience; a room in hell with only your name on the door." I was drowning in my own depression and anxiety and didn't know what to do.

I am forever thankful that this is not where my story ended. One day in late April I was asked by a friend, also a medical student, to come over to her house for supper. When I arrived, she took one look at me and asked, "What's wrong?" and I broke down sobbing and was finally able to share with someone how desperate and alone I felt.

If it wasn't for her and another friend's support, I would not be where I am today. They not only helped me to contact the people I needed to that night, but also ensured I got the help I needed. They didn't judge me, they didn't rationalize or normalize my behaviour. They saw that I needed help and I wasn't capable of doing this on my own. Most importantly, they finally got through to me that it is okay to not be okay.

They helped me to contact the supports available in the College of Medicine, and a psychiatric nurse who specializes in helping medical students, residents, and physicians with personal struggles. The very next day this nurse called me and had me come into her office, where she heard my story, recognized I was in crisis, and got me a same-day appointment with a family doctor. He wrote a referral to a psychiatrist, a note for a leave of absence from school, and I was started on medication.

The most surprising thing to me was how much people cared once I opened up and explained how much I was struggling. I was able to take a week off school without penalty and make the shifts up at other times. My friends made me supper every single night, and other friends showed up unannounced. They knew I would say no if asked, but that they should be there anyway. My mom and dad called me every single day, came and cleaned my place, and got me out of the house and smiling. This all occurred in April, but it wasn't until July that I started to feel like myself. Exercise, eating healthy, and spending time with supportive people I love went hand in hand with the medication to bring me back to a place where I felt like myself.

A wise doctor used a metaphor that has stuck with me: "The medication is the bicycle, but you have to push the pedals." Especially with depression, I felt that you go through the motions for a long time until the negative voice in your head shuts up for five seconds so you can take a single breath.

I don't believe that my struggles with mental illness started in my third year of medical school. I am a Type A overachiever with no experience of failure, and have been that way for my whole life. I think many factors predisposed me to my struggles, and the enormous demands medical school placed on me exhausted my coping mechanisms to a point where things started manifesting in disease patterns. The fear of failure, of being inadequate, and never knowing enough can be suffocating. It is what makes many people succeed, but can also be our worst Achilles' heel. With that, I truly believe there is a difference between the necessary stressors of medical school, or, in a larger context, life, and experiencing the feelings of being overwhelmed with unnecessary anxiety, burnout, or depression.

I've come to see the more I share my story, the harder it is for other people to keep from sharing theirs. The number of peers, family members, and acquaintances who have shared their stories with me since this happened has been absolutely shocking. In talks I have given to medical students, consistently over 50 per cent of the audiences have identified as having some form of mental illness.

The best thing that happened to me in medical school, and the best thing I did for myself, was to open myself up, to tell people what was wrong when they asked. I got help early, before I registered on the college radar by failing a test or getting a poor evaluation. Maybe it was courage, but mostly it was being at rock bottom and willing to admit it.

What does this mean in the context of mental health? Why is this relevant? I think it is relevant because medical student wellness is paramount. Resiliency prevents burnout, improves patient care, and directly improves quality of life. Patterns that develop as a medical student may last throughout one's career. To admit weakness, ask for help, and reflect on your own wellness means having the courage to be imperfect, and the compassion to be kind to yourself first and then to better be able to show compassion for others. I think the earlier this is recognized, the better we as a community will see more compassionate and understanding physicians, less mental health stigma in the health care system, and improved quality of life for all who are touched by mental illness.

Despite my struggles, difficulties, failures, and successes, I had a wonderful medical school experience. I learned more about myself than I ever thought possible and have grown into a person I probably wouldn't recognize when I first started medicine. I realized mental health is something we need to start talking about if we are ever going to find a cure or be able to relate to our patients on even a remotely holistic level. I am now completing my first year of a residency in psychiatry at the University of Saskatchewan, College of Medicine. I believe my own experience with mental illness is uniquely tied to this decision. I now recognize my true calling and passion is in breaking the stigma and silence surrounding mental illness.

Caring for the Young Adult Child
with Mental Illness

Sheila Morrison

When your babe is sick and you can't get the help you need, you turn into a ferociously protective mother. I did.

I will tell you what it is like to be mother and caregiver to a young adult child with mental illness. What is true for me may not be so for you. Take only what helps.

My daughter was an easygoing, happy, intelligent, funny, talented girl who became a little sad in her eighteenth year. The next year she became depressed after her grandmother – my mother – died tragically. A few months later she developed a severe unrelenting (and undiagnosed) psychosis and within a year was admitted to hospital. She was medicated, did not respond, and was sent home with a diagnosis of "behaviour problem" for which we parents were blamed. My protective role was born.

A few days later she was readmitted to hospital and suffered many indignities (rough handling, fractures, unkind words, drug side effects) and remained there because she needed twenty-four-hour care. Seven years later, and still in hospital, she was diagnosed by a smart young doctor as having Micro-deletion 22q11.2 Syndrome (known as 22q), relatively unknown to most physicians. We learned that 22q has over 180 signs and symptoms (such as organ deformities and developmental delay) and that 25 per cent of those children go on to develop mental illness. And for our daughter, the psychiatric illness was the main feature. Had she also had, say, a heart deformity or palate deformity, there is a slight chance her diagnosis might have been picked up earlier. Another difficult eight years of hospital life followed the diagnosis.

When she was deemed stable enough for discharge they recommended, to our horror, a locked institution. We took her home. My professional paid working days ended and I started my new life as a full-time caregiver.

Today, seven years after being discharged, our daughter is content, mostly joyful, occasionally sad. The psychosis is gone. Her sense of humour is back, she has learned to be empathetic and thoughtful, she has many skills, and she is very grateful for many things. She missed many developmental landmarks (mainly social) in those fifteen years, but she is a delight once again.

My role as a formal caregiver really began when she first became sad. I had to relinquish that role somewhat when she became an in-patient, but when the system failed us I gradually pushed my way into becoming a member of her care team. By the time she was discharged, I knew what still had to be done and was happy to bring her home.

Protective mothers have much in common, but we also bring our own unique experiences to the job. I was very lucky in that regard. During my first decade as a new wife (and before kids), I taught school in remote villages in West Africa. My husband and I had learned how to be a team while dealing with tough situations, such as learning to live with very little and unsafe water, no electricity, no teaching tools, and cultures that were foreign to us. When a cholera epidemic swept through West Africa, we learned, as clinic volunteers, how precarious life can be. We also learned each other's strengths and weaknesses and cemented our relationship. Little did we realize how important that would be in later years when we were frustrated by the problems in mental health care. Many marriages fail in the face of mental illness; our early experiences had solidified ours.

In the next two decades, as a physiotherapist working with patients who lived with depression and chronic pain, I learned what was later to be the most important lesson as regards my daughter's rehabilitation: everyone has a starting point, and learning how to move forward involves identifying steps that are small enough to be achievable and guarantee success. The other advantage I had was this: when my daughter became an in-patient, I had an understanding of how hospitals work, an ability to read and interpret a chart, to do an assessment, and to write reports – skills that not all parents are lucky enough to have. What I did not have, however, was an understanding of how mental illness is diagnosed and an appreciation of how fraught with problems the mental health care system is.

I cut back my working hours and changed careers again, moving to a private company where I taught reading and writing skills to adults and children who either had not learned to read or had failed to do well with the usual remedial programs. The success rate of the program was phenomenal and once again the key was to recognize the starting point, offer small blocks of easy learning, and reward, reward, reward.

Identifying and rewarding those small steps is crucial in any rehabilitation process. There is no room for negativity and criticism. It sounds very simplistic and common sense, but to my dismay this approach was rarely taken in the clinical setting. My own physiotherapy colleagues, frustrated by the lack of progress in patients with chronic pain, would say, "They have to want to get better." In the psychiatric wards, the stigmatizing response to my daughter's failure to join in rehabilitation tasks was, "She won't take part in our programs." Such attitudes kill potential in patients. They brought out the protective mother in me.

That's not a bad thing. In the beginning of our ordeal I was hurt and angry. I was looking for a fix, or at least a diagnosis that made sense. Initially I lashed out at staff who hurt my daughter, which accomplished nothing. I turned to the media, with the result that she was moved to another facility. I also joined hospital and community committees who were seeking to improve the system and there I found allies who connected me to resources. The most important of those resources were people in the community who lived with mental health issues and were functioning well and able to talk about their experiences. They became my new circle of friends. I researched, became a writer and public speaker, and spent time with my daughter and her team every day.

I like to think I had some small impact on the

way mental health care is delivered in my province, but my biggest achievement has been in nurturing my relationship with my daughter after she got home so that she could feel safe and capable. To me, she was not someone with "paranoia" and "poor social skills" who needed to interact more. She was a young woman who preferred to be at home. Once a great baker, she could no longer interpret and follow a recipe. But she could slap frosting on a cupcake and share the cake with her dad. And we could celebrate that accomplishment with words and smiles. She gradually took on additional small kitchen tasks. Within a couple of years she was able to have her own dessert catering business for special events.

To me, she was not someone who was unable to walk half a block and shop independently for groceries. She was a young woman who liked to sit in the car and listen to the radio while waiting for me to shop. I told her how happy I was to have her company. One day she decided on her own that she would accompany me for a five-minute errand. Step by step we built on that skill. A year later she was able to walk away from me in the store, find items, and interact with grocery staff.

At first some of her ideas of what she wanted to do seemed unrealistic and unachievable. I discouraged her, not wanting her to fail. When she accused me of throwing up roadblocks, I remembered something I had learned in improv theatre class: just say "yes!" to whatever is offered. I began to say, "Good idea. Go for it!" to every suggestion and discovered two things. One, she sometimes figured out a way to do something on her own despite my unspoken doubts, and two, sometimes she came to the realization by herself that her goal was unattainable and chose another. Either way I praised her thought processes and achievements.

Restaurants were a challenge. Unable to enter a restaurant because of auditory hallucinations and feeling unsure of how to behave and interact, she would sit in the car and wait for a takeout. We made it fun with many picnics. These days we still occasionally do takeouts, but more often than not she is now the one to suggest going into a restaurant for a sit-down dinner. In the beginning she would take writing and art materials in with her to have something to focus on. At first she often left before the food arrived and sat in the car. Now she is happy to sit and chat and converse with wait staff and she can enjoy a meal.

I had to dig deep to find my best self. I found it one night when I was sitting quietly beside her as she groped her way through deep despair. No words would help and because I didn't know what to do I just sat there silently in the dark, close to her, for a very, very long time, breathing slowly and deeply. When she was finally able to talk, she whispered, "How do you do that?" "How do I do what?" "Just sit there and be with me. Thank you." Sometimes my words are not the best that I can be. But just being there in silence can be profound.

I know now that diagnosing a mental health condition correctly and coming up with an effective treatment plan is often difficult and sometimes impossible. I know too that I had a lot to give because I know the person beneath the psychosis and I know her starting points. A camera helped my daughter use her eyes to explore a world that had become frightening. A service dog gave her a non-judgmental soul that never criticizes, only loves her. Having a music teacher who didn't mind teaching for five minutes or two hours in our home gave her the freedom to be able to say, "That's all I can do right now" with no repercussions, just praise for what she had accomplished. It is with a sense of awe that I watch my daughter's recovery and realize just how much potential there is for the brain to change, given the right circumstances.

Goodbye, Mamale

Esther Kohn-Bentley

"Mamale, you're so beautiful!"

And she is, to my eyes. Her ninety-seven-year-old skin is amazingly smooth, her cheeks are naturally rosy, and her white hair, held back with clips, frames the love that still shines from her warm brown eyes.

My mother is beautiful to me, despite her withering frame, despite the pacemaker that now stands out in 3-D on her bony chest, despite the red and black bruises that cover her arms and legs, records of her battles with the bed frame and the toilet.

My mother will always be beautiful to me, even with "mixed dementia" (Alzheimer's and vascular) that makes it increasingly difficult to communicate with her. I visit her a few times each week at the wonderful long-term care home she's lived in for over a year. My brothers and I tried hard to keep her and my dad in their apartment, but because both had dementia, it got too difficult, even with lots of extra help. So swallowing our feelings of guilt and helplessness, we moved them into care. My dad died six weeks later.

But my mother carries on. She will never be cured; she'll never improve. It's a disease that progresses in only one direction. So there is none of the hope that normally goes with visiting someone in a hospital-like setting. There's no planning for when she gets out, since she never will. That fact is always in the air, heavy and sad.

My parents were Holocaust survivors from Poland. They went through hell during the war, losing most of their families. Through sheer guts and ingenuity, they managed to survive. After the war, they were asked to drive a truckload of Jewish war orphans to a Red Cross refugee camp in southern Italy, and that's where I was born. They lived in the camp for a few years, learning Italian and some English, and preparing to immigrate to Canada.

The war was always present as my brothers and I grew up. We lived with the stories of horror, close calls, losses that my parents and their survivor friends talked about always. Being children of Holocaust survivors meant that we suffered then, and still do, from vicarious PTSD, survivor guilt, and flashbacks and nightmares of events that weren't even ours.

There isn't a time with my mother, even today, when all of that isn't there in the room with us. The questions linger, like fog, over the smiles and kisses. How could this have happened? How could such evil have existed? How did my parents create a family and a good life for us after going through so much? How can I make up for what they went through?

That last question has guided my life since childhood. I have always tried to protect them from bad news, get them quick medical help when they needed it, tried in fact to defend them against anything negative that might come their way.

And now, I've hit a wall I can't break through. There was nothing I could do to stop this terrible dementia from taking my dad's life, and there is nothing I can do now to keep my mother from dying of it. I see her decline every time I visit, and I'm helpless.

Here's what a typical visit looks like these days. I enter her room a little anxious, not knowing how she'll be. I find her in bed, scrubbing her lovely crocheted blanket, grinding her teeth with the effort and determination to get it clean. I say, "Hi!" in as enthusiastic a way as I can muster, and wait for some glimmer of recognition to take hold. It's taking longer and longer for that to happen. But eventually she still does reach that point, and smiles happily. When will I lose even that? When will she no longer recognize me? I think that then my heart will be truly broken.

I watch as she keeps declining. Even a couple of months ago, when I visited, she would light up with recognition, and open her arms for hugs and kisses. Then, she could still speak a semi-comprehensible mix of English, Yiddish, and Polish, the language of her childhood. I might even throw in some Italian and she would respond. Now, she struggles to speak in any language. I want so much to understand what she is trying to communicate. Sometimes I think I have it, but less and less frequently.

My mother and I have always been close. I've loved and depended on her for safety and support for most of my seventy years. I still think of calling her every day at around five o'clock to check in on how our days have gone. I can't do that anymore. She hardly knows what to do with a phone. She's no longer able to speak or hear me, though I shout into it, still hoping for a little of what I came to depend on – her loving care, her friendship, her encouraging words.

Even when we're together and we can't talk, I do the one remaining thing I can. I move on to singing. It's true what they say: music really is the last remaining ability for people with Alzheimer's. My dad loved music right up until his last day. That's why, while he was dying, my nephews stood around his hospital bed and sang him out with ancient Hebrew songs, as I sat beside him, held his hand, and cried.

My mother still remembers most of the words to the soulful Yiddish and Hebrew songs of her youth: *"Oif'n pripetshik, brent a fayerl, un in shteib iz heys."* So we sing together, and hand-dance, and I watch as broad smiles lighten up her lovely face. It's all I can do now, to make her life better. I have gradually come to know and accept that the wall is there, that there are concrete limits to what I can do as her daughter now. Letting go of hope, of the possibility that I can stop or even reverse this merciless disease, is one of the hardest things I've ever had to do.

People say I'm lucky to still have my mother at my advanced age. I went through a time during the last eight years when I smiled outwardly, but said to myself, "You just don't understand how hard this is. You don't see the time I spend, the worry, the middle-of-the-night phone calls, the total exhaustion. I'm not lucky at all!"

But as I've walked further on this journey with my mom, I've come to feel genuinely fortunate. I'm not worried about her care or her safety now that she is in a long-term facility. I treasure my visits with her, singing, gently holding her bruised hands, brushing her thinning white hair, loving her up while I still can. I so appreciate the chance to be comforting when she's agitated, helping calm her, feeling I can still do some small things that give her happiness.

I know the day will soon come when that won't be possible any more, when I will be faced with the challenge of really letting go of my beautiful Mamale. I can't imagine what that will be like for me. But for now, I keep my attention on the love we still share, and I appreciate every precious moment I still have with her.

My Mother's Hands

Marty Hamer

1

I will never forget my mother's hands that Friday night. It all happened so fast.

Long day. Friday. Work seemed endless. I watched the clock all afternoon as the minutes came and went – and when four o'clock finally arrived, I couldn't get out of there fast enough. No long goodbyes today. I grabbed my coat, my purse, and I ran. Straight home. Boiled the kettle and collapsed in front of the TV.

Suddenly the phone rang. And I had to answer it. It's my unwritten rule. "Hello," I spoke into the receiver. "Margaret, it's Dad," he said. "We're at the hospital." I was shaken. I grabbed my keys and ran.

It's funny how a drive like that becomes a blur. You have no recall. You do all the right things. Look right. Look left. Stop at stop signs and red lights. You navigate a parking space. And suddenly you "wake up" and you're there. Pumping change into a parking meter – your breath coming in short gasps. You don't know how you got there. And you don't know what's coming next.

When I found them she was in a bed in Emergency. She couldn't hold her train of thought. Words flipped through her mind and flowed from her lips like marmalade. All bits and pieces of things mashed together. "I am where? Your father's with? Did he ... Did he ... When?" I spoke softly to her. I comforted her and held her hand. I told her quiet things again and again. "It's okay. We're both here, Mom. It's alright." But it wasn't alright.

The wild look in her eyes was soon replaced with a vacant stare. She didn't see us and they asked us to leave. They would run some tests. I held his hand as we moved to the waiting room. It was not a nice place. Dirty and cluttered. And filled with faces. Too many faces. Some silent. Some confused. And all like us – shell-shocked – all lost and afraid. One moment life was normal. Regular. And then something slipped, crashed, broke and fell away and now we were here – a band of strangers – all lumped together in this Neverland. Sitting. Pacing. Waiting. What else could you do? The magazines were damaged. Their covers were gone. Pages were missing. You might start a story and find there was no end. Page seven was ripped away. Not that you could read anyway. The stress of waiting in a crisis robs you of the ability to read.

But your focus remains sharp. I counted the tiles on the floor. There were seven chipped tiles in the ninth row from my chair. Their black and grey pattern was designed not to show the dirt. It wasn't working. One fluorescent tube in the bank of lights overhead was burned out. It hummed.

My father managed to tell me she'd been fine. Was tired after her tests yesterday but in good spirits. She ate a good lunch, watched some TV, and then – late in the afternoon – she suddenly collapsed on the floor. That's when he called me. And now here we were. What else was there to say?

We watched and waited. An hour passed and nothing. No news. Just people coming and going through those impenetrable doors. Distant voices calling over the loudspeaker. Dr. So-and-So ... come to Emergency. And then finally a nurse came out. Spoke our name. Invited us back to her side.

When I saw her again, I couldn't believe so much destruction could happen in such a short time. She was strapped to the bed. Wires and tubes everywhere. They were calling a priest on the loudspeaker. I was calling my brothers on a pay phone. Telling them to get here quick. ET, phone home.

Somewhere between 4:30 and 6:00 p.m. my mother had been invaded. Or traded. She was no one I knew. No one I recognized. Swollen and bloated, her neck had vanished. There was puffy tissue where her face had been. This must be a disguise. Where was the makeup man? When was the curtain call? How had I missed so much of the script? Eighty-five minutes. I had been in that waiting room eighty-five minutes. What was happening? I turned to ask the director, "What act is this? What page?" But there was no one to help me. I could not find my place. I could not follow along.

My darling mother – old and frail – had suddenly transformed into a monster. Unrecognizable. Breathing laboured. Loud and raspy. Cheeks puffed and swollen.

Eyelids twice their size. She'll never make it, they told me. There was so much damage.

I sat by the bed. Machines whirred and beeped. Green lines formed on the blue screen rushing rapidly along. Sometimes up. Sometimes down. Falling, falling. Flat, flat. And then jump. Jump. My own heart skipped a beat. I longed for something familiar. Something I could hold on to. One small thing that still contained the essence of my mother. And there at her side tucked quietly under the crisp white sheet I found her hand. It was a hand I recognized. A hand I knew as well as I knew my own name. And I took that hand in mine and I held on for dear life.

2

My mother and I were always connected. As if an invisible cord ran from her heart to mine tying us together. So many times I would reach out to call her – my hand suspended just above the phone in my kitchen – when it would ring. "Hello Margaret," she'd say. And I would smile.

But after the falls and the medical emergencies and the endless forgetting, she phoned less often. Couldn't remember my number. And the responsibility on my father was impossible.

When I moved my mother into the nursing home around the corner, I asked that she have a room on the north side of the building. I asked this because I wanted to climb the stairs in my home and look out my bedroom window – every night – to see if her light was still on. This was a small comfort in our ever-changing world.

My mother now lived in one room. On a locked

ward. Facing north. She wore diapers and slept in a bed with sides. She moved slowly in a wheelchair and although she was able to get around, she never knew where she was going. But we were lucky. Through all this she never lost her warmth and her caring nature. "Smiling Mary" they called her on the fifth floor.

Civility dropped away when she was frustrated. Proper language was going and the correct use of cutlery was a skill she could no longer manage. Her blouse was stained with soup, her slippers were scuffed, and her clothes often belonged to someone else. We put tags on everything but that didn't matter. When you don't know what belongs to you anymore, you can't keep hold of the things that are important.

My mother was slipping away. Every day. But I clung to the things we had. Like the balloon game.

Randy stumbled on it. It was her birthday. He tossed a red balloon to her and she hit it back to him. Her face lit up as he hit it back to her again and a communication was born. A wordless discussion in bright red made up of smiles and laughter. We played this game often after that.

It wasn't that my mother couldn't talk. She could. It was just that her life was so small there was little left to say. "How was lunch?" I'd ask, attempting conversation. "What was for dinner?" But she couldn't remember. We read the menu by the spatters on her shirt. Sometimes she would tell me about things she'd done that day – planning a party or going to a dance – but these were just dreams and confused memories. "Remember when we were kids," she once said, reaching for my hand, and I choked back a sob. She didn't always know who I was. Or where I fit in. But she knew that I was special. That I loved her. And she loved me. I held on tight – content in the fact she was still with me. But sooner or later I'd have to let go.

On the day they took her to the hospital for the last time I was out of town. An afternoon jaunt. A visit with friends. She was rushed in around noon. In an ambulance. When I arrived it was long past dinnertime. Her supper tray was cold. Untouched. I fed her vanilla pudding. "Mmmm ... good," she smiled after several small bites. A doctor came in, an intern in tow. "Can we listen to your heart?" he asked. My mother nodded yes. She trusted doctors. Felt safe in their care. They loved to listen to her heart and she let them. Rheumatic fever as a child had damaged her valves – caused problems throughout her life – but it left her with an unusual heartbeat. Everyone came to hear it.

The young intern leaned in, placed his stethoscope on her chest, and listened intently. He moved the metal disc and listened again. I watched his eyes light up. His fingers travelled to her throat – to the pulse beating in her neck – and again he moved the stethoscope. "It's amazing," he told me, his eyes bright. "Your mother has a wonderful heart." I smiled from the other side of the bed. I knew more about my mother's wonderful heart than any doctor ever could.

The next morning my mother's wonderful heart beat – one last time. And then it stopped. She was all alone. There was no one to call her back from the edge. I imagine her spirit flew off gracefully, joyfully towards the heaven she believed in for all of her life. I hope it was there for her when she arrived.

Tonight my mother's hands are folded on her chest. They are as cold as stone. Her smile is stretched tight across her face. My family and friends help me through this long night and as I climb the stairs to my bed and look out my window facing south I cry. My mother's room is dark. Her light has gone.

In time – when the sadness passes – I will see that her light has taken up residence in my heart. It will shine in my life and I will feel her beside me every time I work in my garden. The flowers she gave me continue to grow and bloom. And I see her smile always in my children's eyes.

3

Suddenly without warning, I looked down and there they were, folded in my lap: my mother's hands.

She had long ago given up using them. She had forgotten how, just like she's forgotten her address, my name, and the lifetime of memories we've shared. Senility, dementia, Alzheimer's. The name keeps changing. The sadness remains the same.

My mother's capable hands forgot how to form a pie crust first. Her once blue-ribbon baking turned to salty hardtack. Inedible. She couldn't remember the recipe. Her fine knitting became endless rows of stitches, repeated again and again, with no beginning and no end. The tension was gone. The rhythm that once held them in place and gave them shape was now jerky. Interrupted. In the middle of a line she lost her train of thought and dropped a stitch, with no hope of ever finding it again.

Her hands, once busy, now flutter in her lap, worrying the buttons on her dress, picking lint from her skirt, pulling at the safety belt on her wheelchair. Those useless busy hands imitate motions and gestures dimly remembered. Those sad hands bruised now from needles, falls, and stumbles have become a roadmap of blue veins going nowhere.

The hands that fuss and flurry in my mother's lap are strangers to her now, just as they are to me, but lovingly I remember her capable hands. The hands that wiped my tears and held my children. Those hands that worked her garden, offered peonies, cultivated daisies, and planted bulbs to the promise of spring. But spring comes no more to my mother. Her vision has turned inward and she sees a world I no longer inhabit.

And then yesterday, on the ends of my arms, attached to my wrists, folded quietly in my lap, there they were: my mother's hands.

They looked so familiar I almost cried. Some trick of time had changed the girl hands I once possessed into the hands of my mother. The baby finger on my right hand is turning arthritically in toward the others as hers has done for years. My blue veins protrude darkly recognizable just below my skin. My fingers arc and ache in the same places hers did.

And when I lose my keys or forget my neighbour's name – just for a moment – I wonder about all the things my mother has passed down to me. Brown eyes, the curls in my hair, and the way I sleep with one foot always outside the covers.

III
Care For (a) Change

The walls are down; the wards are open; but people are still ignorant and frightened of mental illness, and the stigma attached to it still remains.

– Barbara Heaslip
former psychiatric patient
at Enfield Receiving Home,
South Australia (1971)

Introduction:
Women, Caring

Lori Hanson

In this section, experiences of caregiving are reflected on in critical and questioning ways. Here the systems are interrogated, the methods and treatments suspect. Mostly these authors are incredulous, for we seem to fail people as much as we help. The pharmaceutical industry and the medical model drive psychiatric care; research justifies industry and reinforces medical models.

In these stories and essays, the remedies offered for mental health care problems and for health and judicial systems in distress are still partial and incomplete, sometimes even contradictory. But the analyses, reflections, critiques, and recommendations are worth pondering. Some are evidence-based; all are experience-rich.

Madeleine Cole opens the chapter with reflections on an experience that implores us to consider more *Mental Health Care, Not Jail Time* in Nunavut. Hearing her co-worker's story of being locked up for a mental health crisis leads Madeleine to conclude that much upstream and downstream work to improve mental health care needs to be done for First Nations, Métis, and Inuit peoples. We need more than "an apology and short-term programming."

Yvonne Boyer is a researcher at Brandon University. There, with colleagues at the Indigenous Health Law Research Centre, she has embarked upon an environmental scan revealing *Indigenous Mental Health in Canadian Prisons*. That work, recently commenced, already has her reeling. Presented summarily as bullet notes, the stats catch our attention. Deep structural problems lurk behind each of the issues she highlights.

Continuing with the theme of structural inequalities in our mental health care system, Julie Strong takes us briefly into her family medicine practice in Nova Scotia, where she describes changes in mental health care and the two-tier system that has developed over her thirty-five years of practice. In *Mental Health Care in Canada: A Family Doctor's Perspective*, she laments the increased use of psychopharmacology and inaccessibility of psychotherapy to most women. She admits that there are useful roles for medication, but when it comes to addressing women's mental health, we need more trauma counselling.

Safety for women becoming mothers is the issue addressed by psychotherapist Stephanie Irwin. Pathologizing pregnancy and birth has damaged women's psyche, she writes: "society's isolation, stigmatization, and dismissal of the health needs of women and families … contributes to ante- and postpartum depression, and pathologizes mothers."

For a twenty-one-year-old Mary Anne Bain, a

"highly successful scientific career beckoned." But it was not to be. Instead, burdened with childhood trauma and a misdiagnosis of schizophrenia, she spent the next twenty years in the psychiatric system, and then twenty more navigating her way out, through holistic supports. She sums her experience up thus: If Canada can't improve the system, and doctors cannot heal, then at least they should *Cause No Further Suffering*.

"Suffering from depression and getting the flu aren't the same thing, but mental illness is, for the most part, treated a lot like physical illness." Researcher Sana Sheikh takes a good hard look at the medical model of mental illness and the pharmaceutical industry that profits from that model. In *The War Inside Your Head*, Sana illustrates how research funding is incentivizing changes in the DSM (the *Diagnostic and Statistical Manual of Mental Disorders*), in an industry-led direction, away from the social toward a biological determination of mental illness.

In their collaborative research piece, Diana Gustafson, Janice Parsons, Patricia Meaney, and Cherish Winsor use the words of women who are "lone mothers" in Newfoundland to describe how poverty and mental health are intertwined. *There is Nothing Wrong With Me: I'm a Product of Your System* tells us how the women cope with the social stigma, the systemic discrimination, the financial barriers, and the day-to-day struggle of their lives. The researchers conclude that we have to address poverty to address mental health care.

In *The Right to Retreat and the Politics of Self-Care*, we are invited to listen to a conversation between Joanna Brant, executive director at a sexual assault centre, and Rebecca Godderis, an activist-scholar working on issues of sexual violence. Both women wonder how to sustain their energy for this important work over the long term, and both have at times felt burnt out. They take solace in the kinship offered by working on difficult issues together. The conversation reveals their strategies and they arrive at a consensus.

Cathrine Chambers further explores the link between sexual violence and mental health in *Indigenous Women and Sexualized Violence: Therapeutic Interventions and Ethical Practices*. She describes systemic discrimination against Indigenous women in Canada and the ways in which psychotherapists themselves are often complicit in this ongoing violence.

The third section of our book ends, as the book began, with a critique of the ways in which women have historically been pathologized, stigmatized, dismissed, silenced, beaten, and otherwise harmed in our society, including by our medical system. In *The Power of Seeing: Women's Mental Health and the Female Condition*, Donna Johnson describes a career spent working in shelters where she observed the brutality of violence against women and the subsequent labelling of these women as "mentally ill." She calls for a feminist approach that "refuses to blame women or to define their personal struggles in terms of individual pathology." She also asserts that we need more feminist counselling that is "rooted in justice for women. Part consciousness-raising, part sociology lesson, the counsellor makes visible the universal conditions of women's lives, helping women see and liberate themselves from the control and limits placed on them." She is also passing on her feminist torch to the next generation of women, urging us to speak for ourselves and to support the work of resilient women throughout the world.

Mental Health Care, Not Jail Time

Madeleine Cole

Let me share with you, dear reader, a story from Nunavut that keeps me up at night: non-fiction, cruel, and true. I will tell you of a friend of mine whose name is not in the public domain. Her story demonstrates how the health care and justice systems often fail Indigenous patients with mental illness.

We who work in the health field recognize that a person's health is the product of a myriad of determinants, distant and proximal, biological, environmental, and systemic. Some are easy to see and others are opaque. Our life experiences and adverse childhood events, such as witnessing violence, suffering sexual abuse, or being the victim of bullying and racism, can lead the most resilient down a path of ill health.

Let me take you now to Iqaluit, Nunavut's capital and my home, where one day last year, one of my *iqqanaijaqatiit,* my co-worker, exuded an aura of strain and sadness. I reached out to ask how she was doing. She shared her story with me and has permitted me to share it with you.

My friend, the sole earner for her family, was living with intimate partner violence – a frequent scenario I have come across during my practice in Nunavut. I do not know what other traumas she has lived through. She became suicidal. In that moment, in desperation, looking for release from the pain of the life they were living, she voiced to her partner that she wanted to kill herself and perhaps her children, too. RCMP officers were called to intervene – and their intervention focused singularly on her voicing of homicidal thoughts and protecting her children from perceived harm. She was put in jail for forty-two days and had her children apprehended. Full of regret from the outset, she completed her incarceration, met all the conditions placed upon her by the court system, and after three (brutal) months was reunited with her children. When she told me this story, it shocked me to my core that a suicidal woman could end up in jail. While it is understandable that RCMP would have ensured the children's safety, the woman's own mental health should have been paramount as well.

To state the obvious, much upstream and downstream work needs to be done in Nunavut and other Indigenous communities to decrease the mental health burden carried by First Nations, Inuit, and Métis people in Canada. Communities with greater health needs require more resources: that's what equity-based care is all about. In Nunavut, nearly half of adults report having thought seriously about suicide at some point in their lives (Galloway and Saudny 2012). Yet there is no resident psychiatrist in all of Nunavut, nor is there a residential addictions treatment centre. Instead, in the Arctic the judicial system and "cells" seem to be the *de facto* mental health system.

As a family physician, seeing this makes me angry. Indigenous Canadians make up nearly a quarter of the prison population despite making up only 4 per cent of the general population, according to a 2013 Corrections Canada report; often this is due to a lack of mental health services. As the World Health Organization has pointed out, globally, prisons are bad for mental health and are sometimes used as dumping grounds for people with mental disorders (WHO, n.d.).

As well as the need for *more* mental health resources, the people in health care and justice need to reflect the populations they serve – they need to *be* the populations they serve; they need to care more about the people they serve. We need more Indigenous physicians, nurses, jurists, judges, lawyers, social workers, and police and RCMP. And for non-Indigenous caregivers and justice workers, myself included, cultural safety is a long and challenging journey.

My colleague's story is but one of many in Nunavut. Her experiences, and those of many other Indigenous Canadians, are a call for significant system change. Poverty combined with a very specific colonial history provide fertile breeding grounds for mental illness and for crime. Issues such as high unemployment, lack of educational opportunities, substandard housing, inadequate health care and recreation facilities, and in many cases families whose generations are recovering from the deep mental anguish of residential school and other state-led traumas will not get better with an apology and short-term programming. All of us need to advocate vociferously for real change.

References

Galloway, Tracy and Helga Saudny. (2012). "Inuit Health Survey 2007-2008: Nunavut-Community and Personal Wellness." http://www.inuitknowledge.ca/sites/naasautit/files/attachments/2008CommunityPersonalWellness-nunavut.pdf

World Health Organization. n.d. "Information Sheet: Mental Health and Prisons." http://www.who.int/mental_health/policy/mh_in_prison.pdf

Indigenous Mental Health in Canadian Prisons

Yvonne Boyer

In January 2016, working with the Indigenous Health Law Research Centre (IHLRC) at Brandon University, I obtained funding from the Canadian Bar Association for an environmental scan to examine the health status of people who are incarcerated. Just two months into the scan, the research team is alarmed by the statistics and situations we have discovered among Canada's most vulnerable. To illuminate them, the following bullet notes underscore important background and highlight some of the health issues surfacing in the research.

• While Aboriginal people make up about 4% of the Canadian population, as of February 2013, 23.2% of the federal inmate population is Aboriginal (First Nation, Métis, or Inuit). There are approximately 3,400 Aboriginal offenders in federal penitentiaries; approximately 71% are First Nation, 24% Métis and 5% Inuit.[1] In the period between March 2010 and January 2013, the Prairies Region of the Correctional Service of Canada (primarily the provinces of Manitoba, Saskatchewan, and Alberta) accounted for 39.1% of all new federal inmate growth. Aboriginal offenders, who now comprise 46.4% of the Prairie Region inmate population, led most of this growth.[2] Aboriginal people are overrepresented in segregation and maximum-security populations.[3]

• Federally sentenced offenders often arrive in prison with chronic or unmet health conditions. Their health needs are complex and include a higher than average incidence and prevalence of infectious diseases, mental health illnesses, and chronic conditions. Overall, inmates consistently have poorer health than Canadians at large. Health conditions are frequently exacerbated by histories of trauma, substance abuse, or addiction issues. From a determinant of health perspective, it is a high needs population that requires a wide variety of services and supports.[4]

• Since 2005, CSC has spent over $90 million to strengthen mental health services in the prisons. In many cases, mental health issues are treated as security issues, with self-harming inmates being placed in segregation as a way of controlling them rather than providing them with mental health care. Instead of providing inmates with meaningful rehabilitation, they are often making health care issues worse by failing to address them in a humane and effective manner. Tragic stories such as that of Ashley Smith indicate that current mental health strategies are not working.[5]

• Suicide rates are 7 times higher in prisons than in the average population.[6] In a ten-year period (1998-2008), over 100 inmates committed suicide in federal penitentiaries.[7] One reason for the high number of suicides in prison is due to a lack of understanding of the symptoms of mental illness and misinterpretation of behaviours associated with mental illness.[8]

• Female inmates do not have access to mental health supports and services that address their unique challenges (e.g., history of physical and sexual abuse) and Aboriginal inmates have very limited access to culturally appropriate programs/services, and are less likely than other inmates to receive mental health care while they are incarcerated.[9]

• Over the past five years, budget cuts have led to decreases in rehabilitative programs,[10] and a dramatic increase in the number of double-bunking (placing two inmates in a cell designed for one).[11]

• Most federal penitentiaries lack 24/7 health care staffing; access can be particularly challenging during the night shift and on weekends, especially in more isolated locations.[12]

• Transgender complaints at the Canadian Human Rights Commission almost doubled over a 15-year period.[13] In prison, transgendered women are living in all-male institutions – they have to be in protective custody because of ongoing rapes. If they are on hormone therapy, they become increasingly female – but current CSC policy states that with male genitalia they must stay in male prisons and not with the gender they identify with.[14]

Just a few bullet notes from our scan help to highlight the deep structural problems we are uncovering. In summary, health and especially mental health concerns are not being addressed in our prison systems in Canada. Canadian prisons are crowded, violent, and under-resourced. Aboriginal people are highly overrepresented. Women prisoners' unique needs are unmet. Transgendered people are particularly vulnerable. Prisons are filled with the mentally ill, people with chronic health issues and substance abuse issues, and people with cognitive disabilities and brain injuries. Much more needs to be researched and there is much to be done.

Phase 1 of our environmental scan is near completion. It will soon be time to turn to Phase 2. In the next phase, critical questions (interviews) will be asked of key stakeholders such as the Elizabeth Fry Association, the Correctional Investigator of Canada, Corrections Canada, and Prison Health to help provide analysis of these and other issues. We hope to have access to discuss health issues with inmates. We need to ask questions about the transfer or portability of constitutionally protected Aboriginal and treaty rights to the incarcerated. Our goal is to determine whether there have been any breaches of these rights, as this scan leads us to suspect.

References

1. Office of the Correctional Officer, *Backgrounder: Aboriginal Offenders – A Critical Situation* (Ottawa: Office of the Correctional Investigator, 2013) online: http://www.oci-bec.gc.ca/cnt/rpt/oth-aut/oth-aut20121022info-eng.aspx.

2. Ibid.

3. Ibid.

4. Office of the Correctional Investigator, *Annual Report 2013-2014 of the Office of the Correctional Investigator* (Ottawa, Office of the Correctional Investigator) p. 20.

5. Office of the Correctional Investigator, *Risky Business, An Investigation of the Treatment and Management of Chronic Self-Injury Among Federally Sentenced Women* (Ottawa: Office of the Correctional Investigator, 2013) p. 27.

6. Centre for Addiction and Mental Health, *Mental Health and Criminal Justice Policy Framework*, (2013) p. 9 [CAMH].

7. Ibid.

8. Ibid.

9. CAMH, supra note 6 p. 10.

10. Office of the Correctional Investigator, *Annual Report 2012-2013 of the Office of the Correctional Investigator* (Ottawa, Office of the Correctional Investigator) p. 22.

11. Ibid.

12. Ibid.

13. Canadian Human Rights Commission, *Number of Trans-related complaints received by the CHRC – Prepared for the Department of Justice,* (Statistical Analysis Unit – Promotions Branch, 2016).

14. J. Metcalfe, "CSC fails to bring transgender policy in line with international standards." West Coast Prison Justice Society (May 21, 2015) online: West Coast Prison Justice Society http://prisonjustice.org/2015/05/21/csc-fails-to-bring-transgender-policy-in-line-with-international-standards.

Mental Health Care in Canada:
A Family Doctor's Perspective

Julie Strong

I have been caring for women in Nova Scotia for more than thirty-five years. Many changes have occurred throughout the country since I started working as a family doctor. Most significant are the increased use of medication and the transfer of psychotherapy from publicly funded psychiatrists to private psychologists.

Over half my female patients suffer from symptoms of anxiety or depression and many are on medication. It is widely available, since it is covered by both private and provincial drug plans. It definitely has its place. For instance, three weeks ago I saw a forty-year-old woman, "totally stressed out" at work and having constant battles with her kids. She is an intelligent, upbeat kind of person, but with no time for or interest in psychotherapy. After ten days on antidepressants, she reports feeling calmer at work and around her family. I am thankful to have helped.

However, medication does not address why the person is depressed or anxious. Often symptoms that are attributed to depression, like low self-esteem, poor concentration, and sleep disturbance, stem from early childhood trauma. This is particularly so for a woman who was sexually abused in childhood. Medication may help her function at her work, but it cannot address her trauma. For this, talk therapy is needed.

Twenty-five years ago I saw a psychiatrist. A referral took just a few weeks then; now it can take up to a year for an appointment. I became sad when my youngest daughter turned four. I never connected my sadness with the fact that I was four when my mom died after giving birth to my baby sister and our dad basically gave up on life. I asked to see a female psychiatrist, thinking that a woman would be more empathetic than a man. But the psychiatrist sat eight feet away from me, as if I were contagious, and listened impassively to my pain-filled story. At the end of the hour, she handed me a sample package of tranquilizers and murmured something about psychodynamic therapy. I knew I needed healing, but it wasn't going to happen here. Luckily, shortly afterwards, I found a therapist who guided me through layers and layers of forgotten and unexpressed grief.

In Nova Scotia, psychologists charge around $160 an hour and other psychotherapists between $80 and $150. Most national insurance plans, Blue Cross, Sun Life, etc., will cover a few sessions, meaning that only the well-off can afford this kind of treatment. Unfortunately, and certainly contrary to the spirit of the Canada Health

Act, we now have a two-tier system in the field of mental health. People who cannot afford private therapists and cannot wait a year to see a psychiatrist are seen at mental health centres. There they will see a counsellor for a few sessions, receive a workbook on coping with anxiety, and be signed up for a group program. The atmosphere conveys the impression that resources are scarce and people in crisis have priority. Folks who are unhappy yet functioning must make do with what they are given. They are advised to follow up with their family doctor, so they come to me for prescriptions and support.

I have learned that the only way I can be present for, and empathize with, my depressed patients is if I get help myself. I see a psychotherapist every four to six weeks. I have also been fortunate to receive healing from local Mi'kmaq women elders, many of whom are residential school survivors and know much about healing from trauma. Traumatized girls often internalize feelings of shame and anger which later manifest as depression. I wish groups of girls could spend time in nature, with an elder. Healing requires expression of pain and outrage, something our society does not encourage, especially in women, young or old.

I occasionally recite Greek myths to an inner-city youth group. I think engaging the imagination provides a container for painful experience and myth helps us gain perspective on ourselves by connecting us with our past. It gives us a sense of belonging to a greater whole.

I believe we need to widen our repertoire for helping both adults and children heal from trauma, before they develop depression. Medication is useful for short-term management of symptoms, but not for long-term use. More psychotherapists are needed, and their services should be made available to those who cannot presently afford them. We also need to encourage imagination and creativity. Fostering these can help us heal each other and our communities.

Safety

Stephanie Irwin

It is well recognized in the literature on maternal/infant outcomes that maternal physical, emotional, and economic safety greatly increases the chances of healthy maternal and infant outcomes. Yet how safe is it to be a mother in 2017?

For the more than thirty years of my intimate involvement with women and their families during the transition to parenthood, I have witnessed our society's isolation, stigmatization, and dismissal of the healthy needs of women and families. This harmful pattern contributes to ante- and postpartum depression, and pathologizes mothers.

Women's mental health has historically been determined by men. I feel it is imperative that we do not further marginalize women as they struggle with the wide range of responses to the stressors of pregnancy and motherhood. As a psychotherapist, I would suggest a compassionate reframing of women's maternal experiences as "normal" in the spirit of Allen Frances' *Saving Normal* (2013), wherein women's feelings are normal responses.

When women first come to my office, they express overwhelming guilt and profound lack of confidence in the ability to develop and grow as healthy mothers. They are frightened, isolated, and ashamed. Their partners feel helpless and lost and confused. These women are unable to eat, unable to soothe, unable to self-regulate, and they are plagued by obsessive thoughts. They are faced with sleeplessness, anxiety, and a total lack of confidence in their competence as mothers. The stigma associated with ante- and postpartum depression, however, prevents many women from seeking help.

What supports exist for women when they have become mothers? Most women work outside the home, yet the marketplace is still uncommitted to recognizing that the children of employees exist. Just consider how physically separate most child care is from the workplace. I have heard many stories of women being pressured by their managers to continue to work up until the due date of their baby. Society fails to ensure universally affordable and accessible daycare, as well as sufficient flex-time for it. This is fundamentally an absence of real respect for the needs of healthy family functioning. The fear of loss of income/job is ever-present.

Isolation is also a common experience for new parents. The "parent partner" often returns to paid employment within two weeks of the child's birth. And so, the primary caregiver is left alone daily with the infant. Too often the community in which she lives is also empty throughout the day, while everyone works outside the home. Her only connection to other women is perhaps online. "Don't forget to tell them how lonely it is," says a mother of three preschool children. Her parents, who might be a support, are on the other side of the continent. Her partner is frequently unavailable, absent from fulfilling the parental requirements. She feels she is on her own.

Before motherhood, the woman felt competent. Now she is exhausted, overwhelmed, and outmanoeuvred by infants and children. Rather than pathologize her, we can see this as a system failure. I wish to start a lobby to change our rigid, harmful view of what is a normal response to pregnancy, delivery, and postpartum, toward an inclusive, healthy view of women's experience during the child-bearing years. We need more supports for women during their child-bearing years to keep them connected to others. We need systems in place to ensure that everyone has access to affordable child care. We also need to ensure that any woman who is struggling has the means, and courage, to ask for help. Finally, we need to restore women's confidence in themselves and promote their leadership roles. Then, and only then, women will be safe.

Cause No Further Suffering

Mary Anne Ruth Bain

My life has been measured out in twenty-year segments. The first segment was marked by traumatic beginnings, my childhood lost as family wounds were passed on and multiplied.

The next twenty years were swallowed up by the psychiatric system, my personhood lost as I was labelled, drugged, and segregated from society.

This was followed by another twenty-year period. This segment encompassed my recovery from the combined traumas of my childhood and of the subsequent psychiatric treatment.

In my healing, I have been able to reclaim my identity and my dignity as a human being, as a woman, and as a child of God.

Today, at sixty-one, it seems as if my life has barely begun. It is an exciting time, a fruitful time, though fraught with difficulties. I am well-connected to my faith community wherein I have found strength and courage, meaning and purpose to my life, a sense of belonging and close friendships.

Nonetheless, there are serious concerns brought on by my past, extensive psychiatric history, and the long-term health and social effects of drug treatment. The reality of having been cut off from mainstream society for so long leaves me vulnerable and dependent on social services and a health care system that often fails to be kind or sympathetic to a poor, older woman who is also an ex-mental patient.

Could my life have taken a different turn? Could I have found appropriate help, appropriate mental health care earlier? Probably not.

Going back to those crucial and traumatic early years, I did have one notable strength: I was gifted with a fine intellect and an insatiable thirst for knowledge and understanding of the world around me. This provided an opening to escape the crushing burdens of my youth.

In order to thwart boredom at school, I delved into academic books beyond my tender years. My natural ability to teach others surfaced at an early age.

I left the "family" upon being accepted into a science program at a prestigious university. By the age of twenty, while continuing my studies, I was teaching a first-year biology course and conducting groundbreaking research in biochemical genetics. Students and faculty alike held me in high esteem. A highly successful scientific career beckoned.

But my personal life was steeped in inner suffering and I knew I needed help. I could not run away from my past but would need to face it head-on. The science could wait. I sought help.

The day after my twenty-first birthday, as recommended by a doctor from the University Health Services, I checked myself in to a psychiatric ward. "A week or two," the doctor had said, "a safe place to get your bearings." I walked through those hospital doors anticipating the help I had desired for so long. It was not to be.

I was very quickly labelled as schizophrenic and was drugged. Back at the university, faculty and students alike were shocked to find me turned into a mental patient. With one swift diagnosis, I was transformed from a prodigy to a pariah.

As for myself, I was dumbfounded to discover that the standard treatment for someone whose psyche, whose spirit had been so wounded in childhood was to severely numb their minds with neuroleptic drugs. Electroshock was another option. Recovery was not possible. Apparently someone with my condition, as I was told by a treating doctor, was "too crazy to talk to."

As psychiatric treatment continued I became more or less mute. My sufferings from the inhuman treatment were almost unbearable. I will not recite the details here. I know it can too easily be said that having been given the label schizophrenic, I lack credibility.

From early on I have been called to hear people's stories – in hospitals, on the back wards, in the halfway houses, boarding homes, and on the streets. I have listened to the details the doctors refused to hear (or perhaps were afraid to hear). The common truths that run through these tellings are childhood abuse and/or traumas.

My situation is perhaps not unique except in that I did escape the psychiatric system after twenty years. This occurred only because a doctor was moved to wean me off all drugs. He saw me as suffering so profoundly from the side effects of the mega doses I was on that he started cutting back the dosage and then simply continued until I was on nothing (I do not believe this was his original intention). He was adamant, though, that no one could do psychotherapy with a schizophrenic.

Nonetheless, after twenty years I was drug free and slowly my ability to spontaneously think and speak improved. Once more I had the ability, the focus, and the interest to read books. I found my way to a private therapist, a medical doctor (covered by OHIP) who was very successful in treating mental patients without drugs. His lengthy experience in the mental health field proved to him that the drugs used by psychiatry actually prevent recovery.

I was in intensive therapy with this doctor for about ten years. It was slow going at first. My trust in doctors, social workers, in the whole medical system, had been badly damaged by my time in psychiatry. I was petrified of being locked up and drugged again. Gradually, I learned that this new doctor could be trusted. The difficulties which had brought me to seek psychiatric help more than twenty years earlier could finally be addressed.

I also worked with a social worker who specialized in treating childhood trauma (she waived her usual fee). In the latter part of my recovery my doctor's wife also took part – she had trained and worked in a drug-free mental health hospital in England. I came to know the doctor's adult children as well. He realized I had no understanding or experience of a loving family so offered his own as an example. Talking, writing, play therapy, painting, sculpture, and other creative arts were all part of my recovery.

My therapist believed in the holistic approach; the whole person – mind, body, and spirit – needed to be healed. As my time with him was drawing to a close, he helped launch me into the second stage of my recovery, which was primarily spiritual. I searched out my spiritual roots and found my way back home to the Catholic Church. The support and healing I have received within my faith community has made all the difference. I have a life to live and a means to live it.

How is it that I have received all this special treatment? I have neither resources of my own nor family support. Yet I received the kind of personal caring help and love that leads to recovery. Very few people in my impoverished position receive it. But should they not?

I am still called to hear the stories of those who come my way, those who are lost and struggle with difficult pasts – the outcasts of society. And what this next twenty-year segment of my life will hold remains to be seen. I will be fine – but I need to ask for the others:

Has the mental health system changed in any significant way or are labels and drugs still the benchmark treatments?

Today, are bright young women, having survived childhood trauma and/or abuse, still losing their lives to the psychiatric system?

When will the cost in lives and dollars be too high and the system collapse?

Surely Canada can do better than this. And if doctors cannot heal, could they at least cause no further suffering?

The War Inside Your Head

Sana Sheikh

(Reprinted with permission from The Jacobin 2015-07)

Researchers are battling over how to identify and treat mental illness, but the changes may help pharmaceutical companies more than patients.

Suffering from depression and getting the flu aren't the same thing, but mental illness is, for the most part, treated a lot like physical illness. Both are understood through a binary framework that distinguishes between health and sickness, order and disorder, function and dysfunction. This framework – the medical model – treats mental illnesses like depression and schizophrenia as natural, uniform entities that, like physical illnesses, can be empirically discovered and described. Just as you can get the flu, you can get depressed.

The main purveyor of the medical model of mental illness is the *Diagnostic and Statistical Manual of Mental Disorders*, or the DSM, a compendium of psychiatric disorders first issued in 1952 that conceptualizes mental illnesses as "dysfunctions" that occur "inside the head" of the patient.

The DSM has been controversial from the start. Supporters argue that the medicalization of mental illness, as embodied by the DSM, is beneficial for those suffering from mental illness and their loved ones. It legitimates mental illness in the public discourse and undermines pervasive ideas that mental illness is not real or is exaggerated by patients – or that mental illness reflects a defect of moral character or a "weakness of will."

Critics of the DSM have long argued that the medical model divorces mental illnesses from the social and historical conditions in which they arise. By assuming that the cause of mental illness lies entirely within the person and not in society, the medical model and the DSM depoliticize the distress of the disadvantaged and marginalized. At the same time, the business of codifying and treating mental illnesses is also quite lucrative, sparking concerns that the needs of those suffering often come second to the needs of the insurance and pharmaceutical industries.

Recently, however, the loudest critiques of the DSM have come not from the Left, or the anti-psychiatric movements, but from the major players in the mental health field itself. The National Institute of Mental Health (NIMH) – the largest funder of mental health research in the United States and a long-time stalwart of the DSM – has dramatically changed its position on the diagnostic manual over the past few years. Now sharply critical of the manual's validity, the NIMH is calling for the field to move away from the diagnostic manual altogether and towards a new paradigm of mental illness.

DSM diagnoses are limited to be sure, and many of the NIMH's criticisms are right on target. But the institute's alternative vision does nothing to challenge the binary medical model of mental illness. Instead, the NIMH's plan moves the field more closely towards it by arguing that any understanding of mental illnesses needs to be based in objective, biological data.

The NIMH's policy shift away from the DSM and towards a new biology of mental illness did not come out of the blue. It is a direct response to the pharmaceutical industry's failure to develop effective, profitable psychiatric drugs over the past decade. The NIMH hopes to revitalize the state of psychiatric research, and help solve the profitability crisis in the pharmaceutical industry – thus ensuring continued investment by Big Pharma – by aligning the way psychologists and psychiatrists think about, and treat, mental illness with the needs of major drug companies.

The DSM and Its Limitations

The DSM, published by the American Psychiatric Association, is more than just an academic enterprise in psychiatric nosology, the medical science of classifying disease. It is the authoritative manual for classifying and diagnosing mental illness and affects everyone who seeks treatment for mental illness in the U.S.

Only DSM diagnoses are covered by private insurance companies and government assistance programs such as Medicare. So if you're having an existential crisis, which is not a diagnosis listed in the DSM, you had better hope your doctor is creative enough to diagnose you with something like "generalized anxiety disorder" or "anxiety disorder – not otherwise specified," or else you'll be forced to pay out of pocket for treatment. The DSM is also used by other institutions like the legal system.[1] Despite the manual's explicit warnings against reliance on its classifications for forensic and legal decision-making, it is routinely used to determine whether defendants are mentally fit to stand trial or are eligible for the death penalty.

While the manual is pervasive in U.S. institutions, its accuracy in capturing mental illness is questionable. The DSM relies on an algorithmic structure for many diagnoses – to be diagnosed patients must exhibit a subset of symptoms from a much larger list of symptoms.

This leads to high rates of heterogeneity – people diagnosed with the same disorder often look symptomatically very different from one another. Take an illness like major depressive disorder: a positive diagnosis requires a patient to have five out of nine listed symptoms, so two different patients diagnosed with depression may have only one symptom in common.

This variability highlights the thornier problem that diagnostic categories like depression or schizophrenia are largely socially derived categories, not uniform, naturally occurring diseases as presumed by the medical model.

There are also remarkable similarities across DSM diagnoses. For example, anhedonia – the reduced ability to feel pleasure – is part of the diagnostic criteria for depression, schizophrenia, and substance abuse disorders. If you are diagnosed with one disorder, chances are you also meet the criteria for at least one other disorder. So patients diagnosed with a personality disorder (e.g., borderline personality disorder; narcissistic personality disorder) usually meet the criteria for approximately two more personality disorders.[2]

Researchers argue that the high rates of multiple diagnoses suggest that instead of comprising distinct illnesses, the DSM diagnostic system may be "attaching multiple labels to differing manifestations of the same underlying condition."[3]

In the face of criticism, the DSM has been revised numerous times over the last six decades, but serious issues of validity remain, and many experts question whether the manual actually describes "diseases" akin to physical illnesses at all.

Not Medical Enough

Most of the field acknowledges the problems of the manual. But rather than conclude that the failures of the DSM show how limited the medical model approach to mental illness is, the dominant argument today is that the DSM is not medical enough.

The director of the NIMH, Thomas Insel, a neuroscientist known largely for his work on the social behaviours of rodents, has led the charge against the DSM, claiming that the manual's reliance on subjective experience rather than objective measures is deeply flawed: "Unlike our definitions of ischemic heart disease, lymphoma, or AIDS, the DSM diagnoses are based on a consensus about clusters of clinical symptoms, not any objective laboratory measure."

DSM diagnoses use patients' subjective reports of their thoughts, feelings, and behaviours. A major depressive episode is diagnosed by asking patients whether they feel down, hopeless, or worthless (e.g., "Over the past two weeks, have you felt guilty or worthless nearly every day?").

Insel compares this use of subjective experience to "creating diagnostic systems based on the nature of chest pain or the quality of fever," and argues that subjective experience is too fuzzy and unscientific. Instead, he insists, the study of mental illness should rely on objective, observable facts. Oncologists don't diagnose cancer using phenomenological symptoms and psychiatrists diagnosing depression shouldn't either.

With Insel at the helm, the NIMH has rolled out a new research funding program, called the Research Domain Criteria (RDoC), to promote diagnosis and treatment based on objective, biological markers. RDoC aims to "bring the power of modern research approaches in genetics, neuroscience, and behavioral science to the problems of mental illness."[4]

Critically, Insel believes that the NIMH should start from scratch, and develop a new way of thinking about mental illness that eschews DSM categories in favour of constructs informed heavily by the biological sciences.[5]

This is a major shift, and has caused quite a stir in the mental health research community. Researchers at SUNY Stonybrook say, "Our field is embedded in a larger system in which, for many researchers, obtaining grant support is the sine qua non of employment or tenure."[6] Because their careers rely on it, mental health researchers will adhere to the RDoC framework for funding purposes, which ultimately "runs the risk of again forsaking a more comprehensive conceptual model for a reductionist model."

Allen Frances, a psychiatrist at Duke University,

also criticizes RDoC's reductionist account of mental illness: "It is a dangerous myth to assume that patients who meet criteria for 'schizophrenia' suffer only from a brain disease. Contextual forces play a large role in the onset of schizophrenia. A supportive environment, a decent place to live, and therapeutically encouraged engagement with school, work, and social activities are now, and always will be, absolute essentials."[7]

Critics of RDoC argue that the program privileges biological constructs over environmental, cultural, or "psychosocial" ones. This is certainly true, and it isn't an accident.

Bringing Back Big Pharma

"Psychopharmacology is in crisis. The data are in, and it is clear that a massive experiment has failed: despite decades of research and billions of dollars invested, not a single mechanistically novel drug has reached the psychiatric market in more than 30 years," writes H.C. Fibiger, psychiatrist and Senior Vice President at Biovail Labs.[8]

He is not exaggerating. In contrast to the boom in psychiatric drug development of the 1980s and '90s, the industry has come to a standstill, now largely repurposing old drugs for new illnesses.

Major field studies with thousands of patients conducted during the early 2000s on depression, bipolar disorder, and schizophrenia have found variable and lacklustre effects of psychiatric medication for treating mental illness symptoms.

Steven Hyman, a former director of the NIMH, argues that "people suffering with the depressed phase of bipolar disorder often continue to experience severe symptoms even when they take multiple medications with serious side effects" and that for "the core social deficits of autism and the cognitive impairments of schizophrenia, there simply are no effective treatments."[9]

Remission rates for depression are around 30 per cent,[10] and people suffering from mild or moderate depression do no better on SSRI antidepressants than placebo pills.[11] Echoing Hyman, Insel and Scolnick conclude that these disorders are "as much of a public health challenge now as they were a century ago."[12]

Although psychiatric drugs are one of the most profitable for pharmaceutical companies – one in five Americans take at least one psychiatric drug – the lack of promising new psychopharmacological treatments has led the industry to pull back their investments in the field. Forbes reports that "psychiatric drug development has become a dead end. GlaxoSmithKline, Novartis, and AstraZeneca have stopped trying to invent new psychiatric drugs. Pfizer, Merck, and Sanofi have de-emphasized them."[13]

This presents a major problem for psychiatric researchers because, after the NIMH, pharmaceutical companies are the largest source for funding. Psychiatric researchers are acutely aware of this trend. Fibiger concludes, "In order to recapture industry's investment in psychiatric drug development, major changes in psychiatry will need to take place," and that "if we are successful in making the necessary changes, given the enormous level of unmet need left by existing psychiatric drugs, there is no doubt that industry will return and reinvest." Insel and Brady concur: "The business case for psychiatric drug development is not promising" and that "in order to develop a long-term strategy for further development by the private sector, a new paradigm is needed."[14]

This is where RDoC comes in. By treating the DSM as the central cause of psychiatry's failures – and eliminating it – the program aims to spur new research on the biology of mental disorders. For example, very few causal biological mechanisms of mental disorders have been identified – we still know little about what processes inside the body lead to mental illness.

The NIMH blames the DSM for the lack of identified biomarkers and argues that DSM's "subjective" categories have led researchers astray. By focusing on "objective" measures, mechanisms, and biomarkers, the NIMH hopes to regain interest and, more importantly, funding from the pharmaceutical industry. To jumpstart this new understanding of mental illness, the RDoC is now requiring that all NIMH funding applications focus on a limited set of neuroscientific systems.

But the neuroscience systems proposed by the NIMH are grossly inadequate for capturing the complexities of mental illnesses. Scientists who have traditionally studied major depressive disorder, post-traumatic stress disorder, or bipolar disorder are now scrambling to retrofit awkward neuroscientific constructs provided by the RDoC website, such as "negative valence systems" and "arousal/modulary systems" to mental illness in order to attract NIMH funding.

Although the NIMH's RDoC funding program claims to work towards an understanding of mental illnesses free of the assumptions of the DSM, the program maintains the central one – that mental illnesses are "brain diseases" divorced from subjective experience and society's values regarding what is and isn't distressing, inappropriate, repugnant, and morally reprehensible.

Beyond Biology and the Medical Model

The analogy between mental and physical illness is deeply flawed. While it is certainly true that the subjective experience of cancer is irrelevant in its diagnosis, any objective markers found in depression are meaningless if you do not feel depressed. Scientists at Northwestern University are developing a blood test for depression.[15] What if it comes back positive, but you feel fine? Alternatively, what if you are suicidal, but the test comes back negative? It would be odd to conclude that you are not depressed.

Subjective experience is central to mental illness. So while the modest effects of psychopharmacological drugs discovered in the past decade could indicate that better biological research is needed, they could also mean that the key to understanding and addressing mental illnesses lies elsewhere. Obviously biology matters, but the field needs to study mental illness on its own terms, rather than uncritically emulate the logic of the so-called hard sciences for the legitimacy and funding it brings.

Questioning the medical model doesn't mean mental illness is a myth. Far from it. People's distress is very real, and the field can no longer ignore the problems in its current understanding of mental illness. But the RDoC's exclusive focus on biomarkers to draw in pharmaceutical investment will not address these shortcomings. Instead, the RDoC will further strengthen the field's economic and ideological ties to the profit-driven private sector. Its focus on "cutting-edge" neuroscience biomarkers will tether psychologists ever tighter to psychopharmacology and the prerogatives of big pharmaceutical companies.

The RDoC also hurts those suffering the most by ignoring the connection between mental illness and societal structures. As Frances says, "NIMH has had its attention so distracted by glorious dreams of a future research revolution that it has completely lost touch with the desperate suffering of schizophrenic patients in the present. It pays no attention to, and takes no responsibility for, the mess that is US mental health care."[7] Over the past fifty years, the number of public psychiatric hospital beds in the U.S. has decreased from 340 to 17 beds per 100,000 people,[16] leaving poor patients nowhere to turn for adequate care. Many become homeless or end up in the prison system for petty crimes that could have been easily prevented if they had the proper community care. "These patients are suffering greatly not so much for lack of knowledge on how to care for them, but because of a lack of attention and inadequate resources," says Frances. RDoC is part of a growing trend in which state and community services are short-changed in favour of a psychopharmacological model for treatment.

However, despite its deep problems, there is a potential silver lining in RDoC's start-from-scratch approach. The program presents a unique opening for the field to be explicitly critical of its past assumptions and learn from its failures.

It would be a powerful move for psychiatry and psychology to take advantage of this crisis and not only move away from DSM diagnoses, but also the medical model itself and the overwhelming influence of pharmaceutical companies, toward an approach that incorporates subjectivity and recognizes the social and economic basis of mental illness. That would be a real change.

References

1. Slovenko, R. (2011). The DSM in litigation and legislation. *Journal of the American Academy of Psychiatry and the Law Online, 39*(1), 6-11.

2. Scott, S., Pfohl, B., Battaglia, M., & Bellodi, L. (1998). The cooccurrence of DSM-III-R personality disorders. *Journal of Personality Disorders, 12*(4), 302-315.

3. Lilienfeld, S.O., Smith, S.F., & Watts, A.L. (2013). Issues in diagnosis: Conceptual issues and controversies. In W.E. Craighead, D.J. Miklowitz, & L.W. Craighead (Eds). *Psychopathology: History, Diagnosis, and Empirical Foundations* (pp. 1-35). Hoboken, New Jersey: John Wiley & Sons.

4. National Institute of Mental Health. Research Domain Criteria (RDoC). Retrieved from http://www.nimh.nih.gov/

5. Insel, T.R. (2013). Director's blog: Transforming diagnosis [Web Log comment]. Retrieved from http://www.nimh.nih.gov/

6. Hershenberg, R., & Goldfried, M.R. (2015). Implications of RDoC for the research and practice of psychotherapy. *Behavior Therapy, 46*(2), 156-165.

7. Frances, A. (2014). RDoC is necessary, but very oversold. *World Psychiatry, 13*(1), 47-49.

8. Fibiger, H.C. (2012). Psychiatry, the pharmaceutical industry, and the road to better therapeutics. *Schizophrenia Bulletin, 38*(4), 649-650.

9. Hyman, S.E. (2013). Psychiatric drug development: diagnosing a crisis. Retrieved from http://www.dana.org.

10. Trivedi, M.H., Rush, A.J., Wisniewski, S.R., Nierenberg, A.A., Warden, et al. (2006). Evaluation of outcomes with citalopram for depression using measurement-based care in STAR* D: implications for clinical practice. *American Journal of Psychiatry, 163*(1), 28-40.

11. Fournier, J.C., DeRubeis, R.J., Hollon, S.D., Dimidjian, S., Amsterdam, et al. (2010). Antidepressant drug effects and depression severity: a patient-level meta-analysis. *The Journal of American Medical Association, 303*(1), 47-53.

12. Insel, T.R., & Scolnick, E.M. (2006). Cure therapeutics and strategic prevention: Raising the bar for mental health research. *Molecular Psychiatry, 11*(1), 11-17.

13. Harper, M. (2013). Why psychiatry's seismic shift will happen slowly. *Forbes Magazine*. Retrieved from www.forbes.com.

14. Brady, L.S., & Insel, T.R. (2012). Translating discoveries into medicine: Psychiatric drug development in 2011. *Neuropsychopharmacology, 37*(1), 281.

15. Redei, E.E., Andrus, B.M., Kwasny, M.J., Seok, J., Cai, X., et al. (2014). Blood transcriptomic biomarkers in adult primary care patients with major depressive disorder undergoing cognitive behavioral therapy. *Translational Psychiatry, 4*(9), e442.

16. Torrey, E.F., Entsminger, K., Geller, J., Stanley, J., & Jaffe, D.J. (2015). The shortage of public hospital beds for mentally ill persons: A report of the Treatment Advocacy Center. Retrieved from www.treatmentadvocacycenter.org

"There is Nothing Wrong With Me. I'm a Product of Your System" Mental Health and Lone Mothers in Newfoundland

Diana L. Gustafson, Janice E. Parsons, Patricia Meaney, and Cherish Winsor

Lone mothers[1] living in poverty experience daily challenges to their resilience and mental health. Did you know that a lone mother receiving income support[2] is more likely to report poorer mental health than other mothers? Over the course of five years, we collected stories from these women. They told us the cost of parenting alone can cause them stress, anxiety, depression, and other challenges to their mental well-being. Why is that? They told us they feel exhausted and overburdened with having to single-handedly juggle a never-ending list of daily demands. And they do this while surviving on an income that falls well below the poverty line. They can also lack other material resources and social supports to successfully manage the care and well-being of their children and their own health. They must navigate a confusing system to get access to the services and programs their families need. The weight of these burdens is made more acute by the stigma of being a so-called "welfare mother." Such stigmatization is an act of exclusion and these mothers feel marginalized – excluded socially, economically, and politically from the rest of society. Those experiences and feelings of social exclusion have a negative effect on lone mothers' mental health. But we dispute the notion that this is because these women are in some way personally responsible for their poorer mental health or for coming up with a solution for this issue. Joann, a single mother with two children, made this point:

I am used to the system. I grew up in the system ... Everything you have been through, there has got to be something wrong with you. But there is nothing wrong with me. I am a product of your system and you don't want to see what it looks like. That is it. Right?

Her words inspired the title of this chapter and our wish to share snippets from the approximately one hundred interviews we conducted with lone mothers receiving income support in Newfoundland. Their words provide some insight into their everyday lives and how they struggle, some days more successfully than others, to be sturdy and well for themselves and their children.

We, the authors of this chapter, know and understand these stories – not just because we collected them but because each of us has, in different ways, lived this story. Raised by a lone mother, Janice became a social work academic in whose practice and research single mothers have featured prominently. She was the Newfoundland site lead for the Lone Mothers: Building Social Inclusion research project.[3] Patricia was a research assistant with this project and has single-handedly raised her two sons with special needs for over ten years. Cherish was also a research assistant, raising four children alone while completing a degree. Diana, an academic partner on the project, was the lone mother of two children who are now grown with families of their own.

Often when listening to women's stories it was difficult to tease apart physical and mental health problems. At times, we wonder if it's necessarily helpful to know which comes first. What was clear, however, was that poverty was women's biggest stressor, and at the root of their concerns. The duration of poverty and prolonged stress has a direct and profound effect on mothers' physical and mental health. Joann described the stress of trying to feed her two growing children on a limited budget:

You want so many things … The money is just not there. It is just not there. You got two kids that eat like grazing cows and $100 lasts you probably three days. One hundred dollars' worth of food! It's just too much. Too much.

Worries about inadequate nutrition for their children figured large amongst many mothers' stressors. Women spoke often about feeding their children before themselves. Belle's effort to make light of the situation belied her awareness of the injustice:

But there's times you know, two and three days before cheque days, when you tend to run out of groceries a little faster. … And like one day … there was like no meat or like whatever – and I made the kids grilled cheese sandwiches for supper [chuckles]… And Michael sat there, and he had the crust on his plate, and I said, "Are you gonna eat that?" and he said, "Mom," he said, "I'm full." And I'm sitting there thinking like okay, you know that you're living way beyond the poverty line when your kids are sitting down eating grilled cheese sandwiches for supper, and they don't eat the crust so you can eat. [chuckles] … The thing is, you can laugh at it, but how fair is it?

Not having the money to eat a nutritious and adequate diet also contributed to women's poorer physical health, something that might raise concerns for health professionals. Sometimes, however, people in a position to give advice seemed oblivious to women's struggles with living in poverty. Jennifer, who was raising two children, recalled a conversation she had with her family doctor who said,

"Eat lots of fruits and vegetables." But I don't have the money to buy … I don't even know what half the vegetables are at Sobeys [grocery store], seriously. I haven't a clue what to do with them because I've never had them.

Shopping for groceries was a challenge for other reasons as well. Lone mothers told us about the humiliation of paying for groceries with their monthly support cheque while other customers watched and judged. Jennifer's words highlight how damaging this can be to a woman's self-esteem:

People's attitudes, society's attitudes towards people, having to get in line in Sobeys and pull out your blue cheque, it identifies you, who you are. You're an income support recipient and everyone knows it. And that's really, really embarrassing. I'm really embarrassed. … The cashier flicked it around. I was thinking, Jesus, put it in the drawer. Put it in the goddamn drawer. You know? You know. It's just hard. It's just shameful … It shames me.

Lack of money also curtailed their children's inclusion in neighbourhood and extracurricular activities as well as the things mothers could do alone or with their children. Frequently, they felt limited to activities that were free or nearly free, such as reading a book òr doing a 3D puzzle. Rebecca said that distractions like watching a TV comedy were helpful. "I find it really numbs the mind so I can stop thinking about everything." To lift their spirits some women visited a friend or treated themselves to some chocolate. One woman mentioned borrowing a relative's car and going for a long drive and listening to the radio, just to get out of the house.

More commonly, women couldn't afford the transportation or sundry costs of being an active and engaged member of an organization or community group. A cost that many may regard as minimal such as paying for coffee or contributing a plate of cookies is for a lone mother on a very restricted budget seldom a cost they can afford. Such apparently simple things excluded women living in poverty from the simple pleasure of engaging in social activities outside their home. Ellen admitted that sometimes she went to bed to "sleep for two days," just to get away. Her comment points to the creeping sadness and depression that characterizes some lone mothers' lives.

Many women-led families who receive income support live in government-subsidized housing, which is sometimes inadequate and in poorly resourced neighbourhoods that, by design and neglect, encourage crime and social and geographic separation from other, better-resourced neighbourhoods. Susie said of her subsidized housing neighbourhood, "The housing that we're in is just a slum – and it is. Like to me it is." Many mothers acknowledged the humiliation and stress of being forced to live in substandard but rent-subsidized housing in stigmatized neighbourhoods, yet felt they had limited power to challenge this. As Belle said, "You kind of get the feeling you're not worthy. You should think yourself damn lucky when you get a house to live in. Shut your mouth and live with it, type of thing."

Sometimes, however, the only available and affordable rent option was substandard accommodation. Joann lived in a poorly insulated home with drafty windows, mould, and rodents. Her son, who had serious respiratory problems, was at greater risk of ill health in these poor living conditions. She did her best to protect him from getting sick by having him sleep in her room during the winter "because his room has snow inside of it. Like there is ice on the inside of our windows." Her landlord refused to replace the windows, citing the age of the house and the cost of repairs.

Joann was one of many women who spoke about the stress of having children with health problems ranging from asthma, allergies, and chronic bronchitis to autism, serious cognitive and developmental delays, and severe physical disabilities. Access to appropriate services varies depending upon a child's diagnosis and this can create additional worry and concern. Poverty also made it more difficult for women to successfully manage their own health issues such as an unintended pregnancy, arthritis, or stomach problems, and more difficult to access appropriate services to address these and other matters such as a history of smoking, addiction, or depression.

Sherry had a chronic knee problem that required surgery. She applied for a government subsidized bus pass so she could do her shopping, run errands, and do so more safely during the winter. Her application was denied. Twice she appealed the decision and was refused.

Finally, she said,

I just gave up ... I don't have no support from any-body, and I don't have anyone to bring me anywhere. And I had a really rough winter because of my knee. And having to get places and do things, it was really, really hard ... I'm fed up with the system.

This wrong-headed bureaucratic decision illustrates how a woman who wants to be more mobile and to man-age her family affairs is made more dependent and social-ly isolated by the system.

So those are some of the issues women face. But what does it *feel* like to be a single mother living in pov-erty? A single woman raising her children alone faces far less stigma than she did a few decades ago. But that is not true of all lone mothers. Most mothers will tell you they struggle to be a "good" mother but a lone mother who is also a so-called "welfare recipient" faces a set of higher expectations for her performance. And that performance is scrutinized by the system.

Women told us they felt monitored in ways that many of us never have to endure. Ann described with an ironic smile the procedure she underwent to get approval for supplementing her income support with paid employ-ment. "They need to know everything from how many hours you worked to what colour your underwear was, pretty much. It's really, really, really difficult." Women are encouraged to find permanent work and to "get off the dole" but are discouraged by bureaucratic processes when they make meaningful steps toward that goal.

That is just one example of how being a lone moth-er living in poverty is a demanding job. It wears you down. As one woman observed:

There's always some major challenge or barrier that I

*have to try to get around. I can't seem to, a lot of times. I
guess I'm just wore out. It takes a lot of energy ... I've not
really given up but I'm just kind of settling. That's not like
me. ... You can only take so much. I just have a lot of worries and I don't know how it's all going to end. I really don't.*

Maintaining mental well-being under these circumstances is especially challenging.

Rebecca, like many women, talked about how troubled she was after her divorce and the importance of having support systems to help her deal with the challenges
to her mental health:

*Initially I wasn't handling things emotionally very well
either. I was sad a lot. I didn't really think that my life was
anything because the divorce was pretty traumatic for me.
My life had no meaning for me. I had no motivation. I was
suicidal initially. I wasn't bad. It was just thoughts. I had my
sisters, my church and stuff, so I could go to them. Oh yeah.
The mental health crisis centre saved my life. I went there at
least a dozen times initially.*

Lone mothers like Rebecca need a range of resources to help them address an equally varied range of
issues. All need safe, affordable housing and adequate
amounts of nutritious food. Some are leaving an abusive
and violent partner and need protection and counselling
for themselves and their children. Many have legal, employment, and education needs. Some have children with
serious health problems. Some have their own health
problems. How do they manage? How can they be expected to manage?

Rebecca said that walking and exercise were healthier strategies than resorting to her problematic relationship with alcohol. She acknowledged that staying healthy
wasn't easy but she had returned to school. "I don't really

get out a lot. What can you do? You're studying and you don't want to leave your child all the time." Rebecca said that these efforts to do "something positive" helped her cope and to feel healthier. However, when we asked other women how they dealt with their depression, one replied, "I don't!" Sherry, for instance, was struggling with depression when we spoke with her. She told us, "I cry. I cry. I'm stressed out all the time; I'm depressed." The reason, she said, was because "I have nobody. And I have very, very high stress levels actually."

This theme of having nobody and being without a social network was common. Being last on the list and having to manage life's challenges largely on their own contributed to their mental fatigue. The fact that Sasha was single didn't bother her. What bothered her was the feeling of being excluded from everyday life and the loneliness that comes with that isolation. She agreed to take antidepressants. "People told me it doesn't make you feel any better but it helps you accept what you have." Indeed, medication was often the solution that lone mothers were offered and the solution they sought in the absence of systemic changes to a troubled system. Joann laughed as she told us how the endless demands on her as a lone parent were affecting her mental health:

I need nerve pills [laughs]. I really, really do. Yes, I am starting to go through a phase now, I am wore out. Like, everything is just getting on my nerves and being a mom is getting really, really hard and the winter is soon coming. [laughing]

The need to navigate a cumbersome, confusing system added uncertainty and stress to an already difficult life. Women need to be aware of and able to access services that are appropriate for them. Many of the participants reported that information about available resources and services was confusing or withheld from them (whether by neglect or intent). When asked what advice she'd give to other mothers in her situation, Rebecca said,

Get the information. Check it out. You can't understand. There's no way you can cope. You can do it, but it's a thousand times harder. These services are there. People have fought to get these services. They're essential to the mental health and physical stability of people. If you don't take advantage of it, you're losing.

It is obvious to us that women need clear, accessible information. Too often, however, this advice still puts the onus on lone mothers to find solutions to their problems. Sherry told us what it took to get a bed for her child:

When I finally went to Social Services for the bed, they told me you have to be on Social Services for two years. They told me if you go on the system before the child is born, when the child is two, you're on assistance for two years, you get a bed ... I was on maternity leave, now the child is three. It's bad having the child sleep in the bed with me. So I had to get a Sears card, which means a more expensive bed [than] the kind you can get at Walmart, and the bed still fell apart. The drawers all fell apart and [I] had someone give me a mattress ... I just paid it off yesterday and she's five.

Mothers who never married or who were battered by divorce or separation and the ensuing poverty may not, in the face of these obstacles, have the confidence or social tools to move forward with their lives. They may be rendered unable to pursue their education, to get a job, to secure better housing, to feed and clothe their children, or even to imagine a brighter future. And trying to navigate a bureaucracy with confusing and inflexible rules can further erode their hope.

Most mothers reported experiencing challenges to their mental health and well-being. They talked about feeling stressed, sad, broken, fragmented, anxious, and depressed. With few exceptions, mothers receiving income support tended to locate the problem with their mental health within themselves. That's not to say that lone mothers didn't identify problems with the system. They did. But few recognized, as Joann did, that the system was in some ways responsible for their poor mental well-being. What was more visible to us was that lone moms were more likely to accept and internalize the dominant story that points the finger at them and assumes they are deficient or responsible for their situation. Joann said, "I mean, for society the only way that you can get help is if you have a label. They like to label everybody 'cause then it is their way of handling why someone behaves the way they do."

Although Joann was talking about a diagnosis for her son's learning disability, the same bureaucratic logic applies to diagnosing mental illness in lone moms. For women to get access to needed services, they require a medical label. That label is an entrée into the mental health system and lone moms become more eligible for a range of support. The downside is that women are also stigmatized as needy, unable to cope, and potentially unfit to mother because of their poor mental health. And that can put into play another level of scrutiny by the system.

Professionals working on the front lines in a bureaucratic system must be empowered to make individualized decisions at the micro level that make sense for lone mother-led families. Sherry wasn't able to avail herself of services she needed to address her mental health needs because she was not eligible for a bus pass. She told us,

"I've been seeing counsellors and that. But again, because of transportation I've had to stop all that. And you know, it's for your mental health. You need it."

Too often, conservative understandings of social exclusion have been used to tally all the ways that lone mothers are somehow deficient and personally responsible for their situation and therefore personally responsible for the solution. This stigma only adds to their burden, rather than removing it. As an alternative, in 2006 the Newfoundland and Labrador provincial government instituted a poverty reduction strategy built on public consultation. That strategy moved the province from having the highest to the lowest poverty rate in Canada.[4] While designed to reduce rather than eradicate poverty, the strategy acknowledged and attempted to redress some of the structural impediments that have contributed to the continuing poverty of lone mothers on income support. While improvements have been made, lone mothers still experience lives marked by political, economic, and social exclusion.

Unfortunately, the economic downturn of 2016, with cutbacks to programs and services, has disadvantaged women living in poverty who, as we have shown here, have already borne the social and financial burden of caring for and raising their families alone. Having the lowest rate of poverty in Canada means little to those facing the daily challenges of raising a family in poverty. As the province embarks on designing a second iteration of the poverty reduction strategy during a time of deficits and economic downturn, the challenge will be to stay committed to eradicating poverty as a prominent feature of the lives of lone mothers.

Continuing and improved implementation of a poverty reduction strategy and the adoption of an anti-poverty agenda on a national level would do much to improve the lives of lone mothers. A better coordinated system, more flexible policies, and more individualized decision-making on the ground would improve women's ability to move through the system and may reduce lone mothers' stress and the prevalence of mental health issues. Lone or single mothers are, by definition, without a partner in the job of parenting. For these women and their families to thrive, government and other service providers must partner with them, providing the supports they require so that lone mothers are no longer caring alone.

References

1. In this chapter, we use the terms lone mother and single mother interchangeably when referring to the range of women who are sole head of the family (i.e., do not have partners in parenting) without consideration of their current or past marital status, sexual orientation, or gender identity.

2. We use the term income support, rather than social assistance, public assistance, or welfare because that is the term preferred by Newfoundland lone mother research assistants, including Cherish and Patricia.

3. The Building Social Inclusion project was a research alliance established between lone mothers and academic researchers from five Canadian universities and government and non-profit community organizations. The five-year project was conducted in St. John's, Toronto, and Vancouver between 2006 and 2011 and was funded by the Social Sciences and Humanities Research Council of Canada.

4. Statistics Canada, 2013.

The Right to Retreat and the Politics of Self-Care

Rebecca Godderis and Joanna Brant

(Adapted from the original, published September 4, 2015, GUTS Canadian Feminist Magazine)

Our contribution to this book is a conversation between the two authors, Joanna Brant (JB) and Rebecca Godderis (RG). As colleagues we are both deeply committed to providing care to those who have had traumatic experiences with sexual violence; however, we come from very different positions. Joanna is on the "front lines" and works as the executive director of a sexual assault centre (the Centre). In contrast, Rebecca is an activist-scholar who participates in community-based organizing and community-directed research, the majority of which is currently focused on preventing and addressing sexual violence on campus and in the broader community.

Joanna and Rebecca have worked together for over two years on a research project that aims to support the Centre in articulating, promoting, and assessing the feminist expertise of those who work and volunteer with the Centre. This project is essential in terms of providing mental health care because the Centre is known as one of the few local organizations with the capacity to support individuals who have experienced complex trauma. Yet in an era where the medical model looms large and quantified measures of "success" are in high demand, a feminist-centred approach that challenges the fundamental assumptions of these paradigms is subject to scrutiny.

In addition, as an organization that primarily provides services to women, the pressure on employees of the Centre to justify the need for the Centre's existence was intensified within the context of decisions made by the previous Canadian government to dramatically reduce funding for women's advocacy groups, while also amending the mandate of the Status of Women, cancelling the National Child Care program, and eliminating the federal long gun registry, which was partially intended as a measure to help prevent violence against women.[1]

A theme that has come up since we began our work together is the question of self-care. In its most basic form, the concept of self-care can be described as the idea that community advocates, and others who work in the area of mental health (and other similar professions), must remember to take care of themselves if they are to continue to be a resource to others, including to their own families and friends. In our conversations we have felt that this depiction of self-cares leaves us with many questions: How do we undertake "self-care" in a world that is bombarded with gendered versions of consumption as self-care? For instance, the idea of organizing girlfriends to do "shopping therapy" or going to the spa for a pedicure appears to be a common self-care theme. Yet we are personally uncomfortable with how such versions of self-care reinforce highly gendered understandings of what women enjoy, what women are good at, and what women are valued for in Western society.

Less explicitly gendered versions of self-care seem to fall short as well, especially within the context of the intense emotional work that is required of those who engage in mental health care. For example, self-care is often reduced to mantras like "leave work at work," directing individuals to not take their work home with them at night or on the weekends. But when you work in an environment where you must be available to those who are in crisis, and that crisis can happen at any time, this is simply not a possibility.

Moreover, when you encounter moments of vicarious trauma by listening to stories of others and supporting them, the emotional impact of such stories on the listener can be present for days, weeks, or even months. And even when the initial vicarious trauma may be processed, the traces of such stories remain. These traces are what drive us to continue to do the work we do, but they carry with them the weight of pain, sadness, and anger.

In the conversation presented below we work through potential answers to some of these questions. It is by no means an exhaustive or definitive examination of the topic, but we present this as an initial venture into the very real challenges we face with the politics of self-care. At the heart of our conversation is the inspiration we draw from Audre Lorde's articulation that self-care as self-preservation is a revolutionary act. It is an act of political warfare in a society where so many structures exist – sexism, racism, homophobia, ableism, and so forth – that prevent all of us from being well, both physically and mentally.[2] Lorde's concept of self-care recognizes that self-care is not just about individual choices or capabilities. Instead, Lorde demands that we take account of the immense pressures from structural sources of oppression that weigh heavy on all of us, every single day. We invite you to listen in on our conversation about our experiences with self-care and the *right to retreat.*

Rebecca Godderis (RG): There are days that I wake up totally mad at the world. So angry, you know? I just feel that the weight of the enormity of violence against women – of what women face every day – is just too much. And it makes me angry that people can intentionally or unintentionally ignore that, or deny that, and yet it is so clear to me. Sometimes I wonder how I keep going in this world and keep having the conversations I need to have.

Joanna Brant (JB): I think there is a difference in how things are set up for you and how things are set up for me because my environment, in some ways, is more sustaining than yours. Because I have those individual client relationships, I see evidence of positive change in a much more direct way. So a lot of things that you're dealing with are systemic in nature like sexism and misogyny. I see your contact with the students as being parallel with my clients in a lot of ways, and that can be sustaining, but you don't have the agreement with them that I have with my clients: the agreement that we are working towards making things better. I think my contact with clients inoculates me against a lot of despair.

RG: That's interesting. I would have thought that you would have experienced more despair because you hear the incredibly distressing personal stories of trauma and violence that I don't regularly hear.

JB: When I started at the Centre, it was actually tremendously assistive to me to take crisis calls. I was completely able to engage in that work and that felt as though it was restoring things in the world. In contrast, to deal with things like media reports, you are a passive recipient who can't change anything. It is just terrible.

RG: Right, so even for those who are not on "the front lines" per se, the challenges in dealing with the trauma of oppressive systems are still there. That's an important point to recognize for activists and others who work on issues related to mental health, but who may not be doing things like counselling. I think constantly about the structural and systematic patterns of violence against women. I see it everywhere, and I also see the dismissals of those realities.

JB: It really does matter what your base environment is like. In my case, I have two luxuries. One is that everyone at the Centre has a common understanding that the world is messed up, but we also have a collective understanding of why that is, so you don't have to invest a lot of time in translating what is happening out there in the world into the work of the Centre. Also, because I'm the executive director, it means that I have the ability to change things. If someone is badly treated that works with me, I can often do something about that. I can say, "That is not a part of the Centre's philosophy."

RG: That's why my work with you and with the Centre is so valuable. I think what we are talking about is that the two of us working together is really important to make change in the world, but that it is also part of our own self-care.

JB: If you look at what we have tried to set up in our relationship, and look at the parallels to the Centre's approach to counselling, I always say that if someone is having a real hard time, I want them to be able to push back on that by telling themselves, "I don't have to deal with that now. I can take that to counselling next time I go." There is also the crisis line if things really heat up between sessions. I think we have, in some ways, set it up the same because it is an intentional relationship where we schedule time together and are clear that we value the time we have together where we work on the project, but also support one another in other aspects of our lives.

In addition, we have a reciprocal crisis line understanding as well [laughter from both], where if something has just happened and we don't know what to do, we call or text each other. I know I can make a crisis call to you when I am just about to make a really big mistake and I don't actually know how to come back from the brink [laughter]. It is very helpful to have somebody who can actually assist you to interrupt your thinking rather than just listen to you about what went wrong after the fact. Those different points of entrance, both scheduled time and the ability to do crisis calls to someone you trust, end up being really important.

RG: So it seems relationships are central to self-care because they allow us to do our work better in a whole number of ways and to feel okay in the world, but they need to be relationships where there is a lot of trust. It seems that comes from sharing the same kind of approach to the world.

JB: I find the spontaneous connection with people, where there's laughter and it's dynamic and where you don't feel you have to prove anything, is a big part of that. I can do goofy things with people who I know are working hard to make things different, who share the same values, and then it doesn't matter as much what you are doing in that moment of spending time together, it feels like self-care. It allows me to trust people in a different way. You know, a lot of people I really value are sort of "serial activists" [laughter from both]. There is a very clear intention to who they are, what they are doing, and what they stand for.

RG: Very true.

JB: I think definitely part of the trick is also having a place where you can be honest about what you can't do, or having places where you are choosing to show those struggles to someone. There is value in being able to just let it be known that you are having a hard time with something and, you know, that overall I know that you still code me as being competent, which is different than other places where you are always having to assert your competence.

RG: If I'm going to ask myself, "What does the ideal self-care world look like?" it involves having exactly those spaces where you don't always have to be the expert, and you can struggle, but you are still understood as competent. One of the aspects of our relationship that helps to sustain me is that I can show you a moment of panic when I'm questioning myself and still trust in the fact that, like you say, you will continue to respect me, that you think I'm intelligent, and that we are going to continue to have a good working relationship. Those might be some of the most important moments because having someone else to reflect back the idea that "I still understand you as capable when you struggle" allows me, in terms of self-care, to remember that I need to maintain confidence in myself. Of course, we can't always be in that kind of environment but ...

JB: ... you can work towards creating that by schedule and by choice. I mean, part of what we've done is to create opportunities to work together in order to create that different working environment, and then we can extrapolate based on what feels sustaining in that environment to other settings.

RG: Right, so more consciously thinking about which relationships we keep and which ones we do not keep, and which projects we do that will provide the environments that help to sustain us. Then those choices end up becoming an act of self-care. I do think that self-care is too often understood as "What do you do outside of work to make work-life balance better?" And that means separating work and "life" as if there is this clear binary between your work life and your non-work life. Self-care needs to be something that blurs those boundaries. Self-care can be about the choices you make in work life, as well as during moments when you are not technically working.

JB: I think things are often set up as a dichotomous or exclusive terrain for women. There is the mothering sphere which isn't supposed to overlap with the working sphere which isn't supposed to overlap with your love life. If you're not going to create that false dichotomy, then what are the implications for self-care that might be a little bit more than sitting on a yoga ball while you are typing for eight hours? But I keep thinking about the Audre Lorde quote and that there is something about the incredible heritage around that level of activism that seems really unattainable in a lot of ways. I know that's the opposite of what is intended, but I would want self-care to be an act of caring for yourself in ways that make sense to you – even if that's really imperfect and even if it's something that you manage well at certain times and not at others. This is still a revolutionary act. It doesn't have to be a perfect act of self-care in order for you to be a good feminist activist.

RG: Throughout our conversations that is something that has really become clear to me. We don't want to make self-care another thing to check off the list which makes you a "good feminist" or a "good mental health professional." Self-care is messy and it's complicated, and it looks like this because the systems that we are in are so messy and complicated. In fact, when I am in a routine that would be considered "good self-care," like going to the gym regularly in the mornings before work, it also feels like a fake life because it has to be so incredibly regimented. I have to get to bed early in the evening, and I have to have no additional stress that keeps me awake at night, because otherwise I can't get up early enough to go to the gym in order to be in the office on time. It's another form of work that I have to add to my day, on top of everything else, in order to fulfill what it means to be "healthy" and do good self-care.

JB: I've really resisted the concept of self-care for a long time as being another unachievable marker that is used to measure women specifically. There is a funny sort of victim-blaming element there. I remember having a colleague who died after she had a very short battle with cancer. The collective wisdom was "You know, she never really took care of herself" and that was from a community that, right up until she had died, had been very much in awe of her activism, her drive, and her ability to sacrifice her needs for the women, the organization, and the community at large. Then as soon as she died, everyone turned on her in a way.

RG: So is there a different thing we can call it? Something other than self-care?

JB: I think part of what we've been talking about is setting up a life so that it works. You know, setting up a world so that it's not as hard on people, setting up our work so it's not as hard on us, and setting up relationships that can sustain us. When I am starting to feel really depleted, not doing "self-care" is one of the things I give myself permission to do. You know, I'm going to pick up fast food on the way home, I'm going to sit in front of the TV for two hours even if I don't remember what I watch, and then I'm going to start working at 10:30 p.m. when the house is quiet and work until four in the morning because that will allow me to be tired and to go to sleep, and feel like I've moved through enough stuff that it's not hopeless. And in what book does that constitute self-care? It's like the antithesis of self-care in a lot of ways.

RG: So maybe what we are talking about is not self-care at all.

JB: It is a retreat from self-care.

RG: It's the right to retreat.

When we embarked upon this conversation, it was already clear to us that relationships were integral to being able to take care of ourselves. We had also recognized that the expectation of self-care has the potential to place an additional burden upon the very people who carry some of the heaviest burdens: namely, women who care for other women whether these women formally work in the mental health field, are community advocates, or are friends and family. However, what crystalized for us through this conversation was the understanding that having a personal ally who can witness your struggle, while continuing to remind you of your competence and abilities, is irreplaceable. In Audre Lorde's words, it is a revolutionary act. Moreover, our chance to explicitly discuss the politics of self-care has meant that we are now more intentional in our relationship with one another about the need to allow space for witnessing, struggling, and the general messiness of self-care. We plan to have many more conversations about our right to retreat, and we hope this chapter has inspired you to do so as well.

References

1. For more information see Canadian Association of University Teachers website: http://www.caut.ca/news/2014/03/07/caut-statement-on-international-women-s-day-2014).

2. Audre Lorde. (1984). *Sister Outsider: Essays and Speeches*. Trumansburg, NY: Crossing Press.

Indigenous Women and Sexualized Violence: Therapeutic Interventions and Ethical Practice

Cathrine E. Chambers

"When he [the psychiatrist] asked me if I ever saw things or heard things, I told him about my visions ... about the animal spirits that would visit me in 2jmy dreams with messages about my life, my children, my ancestors. I told him that an eagle came to me one night and told me not to be afraid, that I would be protected from the trickster spirits that had haunted my aunt and my cousin. At first he just nodded and looked at me like he understood. Then he started talking ... all I remember is he told me I had schizophrenia and had to be hospitalized right away. I was there for four months. I don't remember much from that time ..." – Theresa, 2009[1]

As a feminist trauma therapist, I often work with Indigenous women who have experienced various kinds of violence. Over the years, I have learned from Indigenous women that while we must confront the pain, the fear, and the terror that accompanies experiences of violence, we are not alone in our quest for healing. I have learned that we are not separate, we are not broken, and we are not "disordered." I have learned that in order for healing to take place, it is essential to go beyond the individualism and medicalization inherent in modern psychology to a deeper sense of connection between all living beings, the Earth, and the Creator.

It is through these powerful experiences of connection and healing work with women who have inhabited Turtle Island for millennia that I have been inspired to investigate more deeply the conditions in which violence against Indigenous women takes place, and the ways in which professional helping has become complicit in this ongoing violence. While I am still investigating how to better support Indigenous women in my research with Indigenous helpers and healers, I offer some preliminary thoughts and reflections for therapists who wish to engage in this work more ethically and effectively.

Colonialism and Violence Against Indigenous Women

The legacy of colonialism and its subsequent racist and sexist policies are inextricably linked to contemporary issues facing Indigenous women in Canada, including social and economic marginalization, historic and intergenerational trauma, and epidemic proportions of ongoing sexualized violence. The introduction of infectious diseases, the experiences of the residential schools, ongoing dispossession of land, and restricted access to traditional economies all reflect colonial legacies (and current realities), which negatively affect the health of Indigenous people. The psychological legacy of colonialism is particularly poignant for Indigenous women who continue to experience the devastating impacts of centuries of sexualized violence. The historical legacy of violence against Indigenous women is apparent in the ways in which Indigenous women's bodies have been systematically exoticized, devalued, and objectified (Smith 2005). Furthermore, the trauma of sexualized violence is exacerbated for many Indigenous women by the interlocking oppressions of structural violence including racism, sexism, and poverty.

Cultural dominance and the idea of psychological "Otherness" have become implicit in the development of treatment approaches for Indigenous women. The dominant biomedical approach to mental health is derived from a European state-sanctioned model of medical practice, which often attributes mental illness to biological causes (Vukic, Gregory, Martin-Misener, & Etowa 2011). Contemporary psychiatry and psychology have continued to evolve in ways that reinforce the biological nature of disease. Psychology now involves the assessment, diagnosis, and treatment of various "neurobiological" disorders in ways that often ignore interpersonal, environmental, social, political, and economic factors (Christopher & Hickinbottom 2008). The modern practice of psychiatry and psychology thus emerge as imperial and authoritarian forces that continue to exert control over Indigenous women in the form of psychological imperialism (Duran & Duran 1995).

Much of the literature on psychological trauma supports the idea of psychological imperialism. Psychology neglects to consider systemic issues of oppression that contribute to the suffering of Indigenous women and communities. Dominant discourses on trauma and healing remain individualistic; that is, they assume a particular relationship between thoughts, feelings, and actions that occurs within linear time, and focuses on individual goals such as greater self-esteem, self-actualization, and self-expression (Vukic, Gregory, Martin-Misener, & Etowa 2011). By contrast, many Indigenous cultures experience healing in more relational and communal ways, emphasizing the importance of familial ties and networks (Richters 2008). We must therefore question the extent to which existing psychological theories can make sense of the pain and suffering that emerge from experiences of violence in non-Western contexts (Pupavac 2002; Summerfield 1999).

The DSM and PTSD

The individualization and medicalization of experience is particularly apparent in the *Diagnostic and Statistical Manual of Mental Disorders* (DSM-V), which is used in modern psychiatry and psychology to identify, categorize, and diagnose various behaviours. Some experiences, particularly in the aftermath of trauma, are labelled as pathological and therefore require pharmacological and/or therapeutic interventions. Despite the fact that limited scientific evidence exists for the biological basis of many psychiatric problems, psychiatry continues to support a medical approach to various problems of living (Szasz 1960). Furthermore, diagnosis happens through processes and frameworks that are socially constructed, and take place in specific cultural contexts. As such, diagnostic categories privilege some voices and silence others; they can vindicate, blame, legitimize, or stigmatize, and are linked to access, or lack thereof, of resources and opportunities (Jutel & Nettleton 2011).

Non-dominant groups, including women, colonial subjects, the poor, the racialized, and the (dis)abled are disproportionately pathologized in the process of psychiatric diagnosis and treatment (Howell & Voronka 2012). In the 1970s, feminists began to critique psychiatry as implicit in ongoing patriarchal violence, citing examples of women who did not adhere to treatment and were subsequently punished (Diamond 2012). Furthermore, feminists have demonstrated that many psychiatric diagnoses reflect particular gender, class, and culture biases, and are often implemented as a way to regulate problematic behaviour (Rose 1998). The contemporary diagnosis of post-traumatic stress disorder (PTSD) in particular has been criticized as failing to address social, political, and economic circumstances that contribute to trauma, thus eclipsing any awareness of the context in which the violence occurred (Lovrod & Ross 2012; Richters 2008).

Far from constituting a timeless, universal experience, PTSD is a relatively recent construct (Fassin & Rechtman 2009). PTSD focuses on acute events and does not take into consideration the larger systemic/oppressive forces that give rise to and even cause the symptoms characterized by PTSD. Although the popularity of PTSD has resulted in greater awareness of the effects of trauma and violence against women, the consequences of a diagnosis turn the survivor's experience into a "disorder" (Burstow 2005). With more and more oppressed people being diagnosed with PTSD, not only are their broader experiences of social injustice, discrimination, racism, and colonialism invalidated, but they are also labelled as "mentally disordered" and subject to greater involvement with psychiatry (Burstow 2003).

Current models of understanding and theorizing trauma should be expanded to take into account both the historic and present-day experiences of Indigenous peoples. The impacts of colonialism, including sexual violence against Indigenous women, cannot be conceptualized only in terms of effects on the individual, as the biomedical approach suggests. Indigenous scholars have articulated theories of intergenerational trauma and historic trauma as ways to explain and understand the legacy of colonialism and how this legacy interacts with contemporary experiences of violence (Duran 2006). These theories are particularly important given the fact that ongoing experiences of sexual violence cannot be understood as separate from colonialism.

Indigenous Approaches to Healing

Despite the dominant nature of psychology and psychiatry, acts of resistance do exist. Individuals and communities are not necessarily passively defined through their involvement with psychiatry; agency is possible (Terkelsen 2009). Indigenous psychologists and helpers have begun to articulate specifically Indigenous approaches to mental health, which often include greater collaboration with elders and community groups and a return to treatments that are informed by Indigenous world views (Broadbridge Legge Linklater 2011). In contrast to dominant understandings of illness and disease, Indigenous paradigms of mental health tend to focus on the connections between mind, body, and spirit; interrelatedness between people, the land, and the Creator; the unification of all living things into a greater whole; and the circular nature of time, sometimes represented by the Medicine Wheel (HeavyRunner & Sebastian Morris 1997). Therefore, depending on the specific culture, healing may involve traditional practices such as sweats, talking circles, smudging, dancing, storytelling, and ceremony (Waldram 2008).

The existing literature regarding Indigenous approaches to healing from violence yields several important themes. Given the assault on the cultural identity of Indigenous peoples, healing often includes a rebuilding of individual and collective identities as well as reconnection with culture (Wesley-Esquimaux & Smolewski 2004). At the same time, Indigenous mental health practitioners recognize the impossibility of returning to a pre-colonial reality. Many may choose to use both Indigenous and Western approaches, such as Coyote Medicine (Mehl-Madrona 2011), which integrates ancient and modern approaches to treating illness, and Two-Eyed Seeing (Iwama, Marshall, Marshall, & Bartlett 2009), which aims to bridge Western and Indigenous world views.

Critical Reflections for Therapists and Helpers

While feminist counselling paradigms have been suggested as a potential starting place for working with Indigenous women, they may still contain Eurocentric assumptions. For example, improving self-esteem through changing one's individual thoughts is an approach often used by feminist therapists to support women who have experienced violence. However, this approach is insufficient in our work with Indigenous women, as cognitive interventions neglect to address relationships to the land, spirit, and community – all of which play a central role in healing. It is important for settler therapists to complete multicultural counselling courses, attend workshops, and learn about traditional spiritual practices. At the same time, although this kind of knowledge is necessary, it may not be sufficient.

Understanding the assumptions we bring to the table is an important part of preparing ourselves for this work, as is an acknowledgment of the power and privilege we bring to our helping conversations. We cannot uncritically rely on Eurocentric viewpoints and approaches, which assume that everything can be known; that there are "experts" who possess specialized knowledge not available to everyone; and that individuals are at the centre of knowledge production.

We must seek to better understand our relationship to land, language, spirit, politics, economics, environment, and society. We must reject notions of certainty in favour of uncertainty, ambiguity, and multiple meanings of events and experiences. We are called upon to inhabit conversational spaces that are often ambiguous and shifting, where events can always be interpreted in multiple ways, and where beliefs, values, and assumptions are continuously challenged.

Despite the best intentions of non-Indigenous helpers, even those of us who are committed to self-reflection, assumptions and beliefs often infiltrate our helping work. Clearly, there is much to be learned. As my research progresses, I hope to be able to further contribute to conversations about how we can better support Indigenous women as they seek to heal from experiences of violence.

References

1. An excerpt summarized from a therapy session with an Indigenous woman in 2009. Some details have been altered to ensure anonymity and confidentiality are maintained.

Broadbridge Legge Linklater, R.L. (2011). *Decolonising trauma work: Indigenous practitioners share stories and strategies* (Doctoral dissertation). Retrieved from ProQuest Dissertations and Theses database. (UMI No. 1324126141).

Burstow, B. (2003). Toward a radical understanding of trauma and trauma work. *Violence Against Women, 9*(11), 1293-1317.

Burstow, B. (2005). A critique of posttraumatic stress disorder and the DSM. *Journal of Humanistic Psychology, 45*(4), 429-445.

Christopher, J.C., & Hickinbottom, S. (2008). Positive psychology, ethnocentrism, and the disguised ideology of individualism. *Theory & Psychology, 18*(5), 563-589.

Diamond, S.L. (2012). *Against the medicalization of humanity: A critical ethnography of a community trying to build a world free of sanism and psychiatric oppression* (Doctoral dissertation). University of Toronto, Toronto.

Duran, E. (2006). *Healing the soul wound: Counseling with American Indian and other Native peoples*. New York, NY: Teachers College Press.

Duran, E., & Duran, B. (1995). *Native American postcolonial psychology*. Albany, NY: State University of New York Press.

Fassin, D., & Rechtman, R. (2009). *The empire of trauma: An inquiry into the condition of victimhood*. Princeton, NJ: Princeton University Press.

HeavyRunner, I. & Sebastian Morris, J. (1997). *Traditional Native culture and resilience*. Retrieved from http://conservancy. umn.edu/bitstream/145989/1/TraditionalNativeCulture-and-Resilience.pdf

Howell, A., & Voronka, J. (2012). Introduction: The politics of resilience and recovery in mental health care. *Studies in Social Justice, 6*(1), 1-7.

Iwama, M., Marshall, M., Marshall, A., & Bartlett, C. (2009). Two-eyed seeing and the language of healing in community-based research. *Canadian Journal of Native Education, 32*(2), 3.

Jutel, A., & Nettleton, S. (2011). Towards a sociology of diagnosis: Reflections and opportunities. *Social Science & Medicine, 73*(6), 793-800.

Lovrod, M., & Ross, L. (2012). Post Trauma: medicalization and damage to social reform. *Atlantis: Critical Studies in Gender, Culture & Social Justice, 35*(2), 40-50.

Mehl-Madrona, L. (2011). *Coyote medicine: Lessons from Native American healing.* New York, NY: Simon and Schuster.

Pupavac, V. (2002). Pathologizing populations and colonizing minds: International psychosocial programmes in Kosovo. *Alternatives, 27*, 489-511.

Richters, A. (2008). Trauma and healing: Cross-cultural and methodological perspectives on post-conflict recovery and development. In Zarkov, D. (Ed.), *Gender, violent conflict and development: Issues for theory, policy and practice.* New Delhi, India: Zubaan Books.

Rose, N. (1998). Governing risky individuals: The role of psychiatry in new regimes of control. *Psychiatry, Psychology and Law, 5*(2), 177-195.

Smith, A. (2005). *Conquest: Sexual violence and the American Indian genocide.* Cambridge, MA: South End Press.

Summerfield, D. (1999). A critique of seven assumptions behind psychological trauma programmes in war-affected areas. *Social Science & Medicine, 48*(10), 1449-1462.

Szasz, T.S. (1960). The myth of mental illness. *American Psychologist, 15*(2), 113-118.

Terkelsen, T.B. (2009). Transforming subjectivities in psychiatric care. *Subjectivity, 27*(1), 195-216.

Vukic, A., Gregory, D., Martin-Misener, R., & Etowa, J. (2011). Aboriginal and Western conceptions of mental health and illness. *Pimatisiwin: A Journal of Aboriginal and Indigenous Community Health, 9*(1), 65-86.

Waldram, J.B. (2008). (Ed.). *Aboriginal healing in Canada: Studies in therapeutic meaning and practice.* Ottawa, ON: Aboriginal Healing Foundation. Retrieved from http://www.ahf.ca/downloads/aboriginal-healing-in-canada.pdf

Wesley-Esquimaux, C.C. & Smolewski, M. (2004). *Historic trauma and Aboriginal healing.* Ottawa, ON: Aboriginal Healing Foundation. Retrieved from http://www.ahf.ca/downloads/research-compendium.pdf

The Power of Seeing:
Women's Mental Health and the Female Condition

Donna F. Johnson

"Freedom and justice do wonders for mental health."
— Phyllis Chesler

A forty-year-old woman tries to throw herself out of a car driven by her husband along a busy highway. Her husband drives straight to hospital where she is assessed by a psychiatrist and diagnosed with "suicidal behaviour disorder," her actions judged abnormal and self-destructive. But what if jumping out of the car was an act of resistance to control and confinement in the home? What if she had decided in that moment to take back her life, come what may? Would a man be considered sick if he risked his life to escape captivity? The woman will be returned to the "care" of her husband, and the label will follow her the rest of her life. If, at a later date, she tries to escape the marriage via divorce, her husband will use her "mental health issues" to try to wrest her children from her. He has the weight of the medical profession behind him.

Years of working with women has taught me that traditional mental health services fail women. No matter how kindly these services are delivered, if the basic paradigm is wrong – and I think it is – women will be harmed. Women are routinely pathologized for legitimate responses to the unjust conditions of their lives. Schooled in traditional models of health and illness, mental health professionals fail to recognize the tentacles of gender oppression reaching into their clients' lives.

There remains tremendous opposition to seeing women as an oppressed group. The oppression of women is so rampant, so old, so embedded in cultural and religious traditions and structures that it is seen as normal and natural, ironically obscured by its very ubiquitousness. It is patriarchy's great achievement over many thousands of years to have so enshrined its principles into everyday life that men and women alike uncritically adopt attitudes and practices that harm women. Gender discrimination is of course not the only bias operating in women's lives, but it crosscuts every other oppression (race, class, ability, etc.), meaning that all women, without exception, are affected by it. The Oxford-trained woman lawyer and the female Dalit cleaning toilets in India both have to manage throughout their lives the indignities, risks, and psychological impact of their assigned second-class status.

From birth, indeed, from the womb, females are treated differently than their male counterparts: streamed into limiting roles, denied full control over their lives, prevented from realizing their full potential. Women are forced to work at lower wages than men and expected to manage the domestic sphere and care for children and families without any compensation at all, beyond being lauded for lives of unconditional love and self-sacrifice. Women are pornographically sexualized, raped in staggering numbers, and regularly beaten, threatened, and killed in their marriages and intimate relationships.

Women who break down under these conditions are routinely diagnostically labelled, yet there is nothing "wrong" with most women. They carry no pathology, no disorder, no disease of the mind. Their distress is a response to the conditions of their lives – overwork, exploitation, servitude, invisibility, lack of support, abuse, threat, coercion, control, violence, unfulfilled potential – all the injustices that go hand in hand with their assigned second-class status. It is the condition of women's lives that is the central problem. If anything needs diagnosing and labelling, it is this.

Feminism offers a corrective to the silence and denial surrounding women's subordinate status. Feminist counselling replaces traditional mental health assumptions with a personal and political understanding of what creates disturbed behaviour in women. A feminist approach refuses to blame women or to define their personal struggles in terms of individual pathology. It recognizes women's strengths and resilience in the face of serious obstacles to their well-being and freedom.

In this concluding chapter I state the case for working with women from a feminist perspective, or rather, restate the case, for it has been made and largely forgotten. I begin, as I do when teaching, counselling, or working with small groups, with my own life. Self-disclosure is a way of liberating experience and emotion and places teacher and student, therapist and client on an equal footing. Like many women I came to feminism in a search for answers to "the unspecified frustrations of our private lives."[1] It is in talking with other women that we gradually come to see that many of our problems are the problems of all women, political in nature and requiring political solutions.

This is not to say that political context accounts for all women's suffering, nor that medication and hospitalization will not at times be required. But women's mental health begins to improve the minute we begin to see we have been duped by patriarchy's fictions into living partial lives. We cease to flounder in mystification and self-doubt and begin the struggle to know who we really are and what we can be.

Beginning With My Own Life

My critical thinking about women's mental health began the day I entered a shelter for battered women. It was the winter of 1986. I was a graduate in psychology applying for work as a crisis counsellor. I was shown into a small office to wait for my interview. On a wall in that room hung a poster that read,

> *In education, in marriage, in religion,*
> *in everything, disappointment is the lot*
> *of women. It shall be the business of*
> *my life to deepen this disappointment*
> *in every woman's heart until she bows*
> *down to it no longer. – Lucy Stone*

The text was accompanied by an image of a woman screaming.

Who would put up such a poster in such a place? I wondered. Shouldn't a women's shelter be a place of comfort and consolation? But something about the poster resonated within my thirty-one-year-old psyche. I began in that moment to understand my life outside an individual and psychological context.

I had recently returned from a year backpacking with a friend. My mother had begged me not to make that trip. "The world is not a safe place for two women travelling alone," she said. "It's a man's world, Donna! You might as well get used to it." We were in fact frequently harassed by men on that trip, and I was sexually assaulted twice, once while asleep on an overnight train in India, the second time during a storm on a Greek ferry. I became seasick and rushed to the bathroom. A uniformed steward followed me in under the pretense of helping me. He molested me as I was on my knees being sick. By the time I was back on my feet he was gone. I never saw his face.

I had been sexually harassed many times prior to that trip, on the street, on public transportation, in a movie theatre. As a student, pornography was left on my desk in the university stacks, and sent to me in the mail. I did not know any of the men who did these things so knew the incidents were not "personal" but a response to the fact of my being female. But what was the intent? To make me fear the public space? To bolster these men's sense of their power and privilege? To reinforce the message that women in public are considered sexually available? I was at liberty to move about, yet there was a sense of being policed. What kind of freedom was this?

The poster held a truth I was in the very beginning stages of understanding. Women hold second-class status in the world, and this plays out in real and damaging ways in our daily lives. My mother was reaching for this truth but never quite grasped it. She knew it was a man's world but thought adjustment was the key to women's survival. She had no framework in which to situate her experience, no community of women to talk to. She talked to doctors. None of them helped her. How could they? They were all mired in the same framework.

My Mother's Life

No psychiatrist ever helped my mother explore the many raw humiliations she suffered in her marriage. My father was a good man in many ways, but he often neglected and insulted his wife. When their first child was born, my father failed to show up at the hospital to bring his wife and baby home. My mother waited and waited in the hospital foyer. Finally, she and the baby were driven home by the husband of the woman she had shared a room with. My father was hungover from partying with the woman next door and had forgotten about his wife and newborn.

I remember the time my mother smashed to pieces the dollar-store ornaments my father bought her as a last-minute birthday gift. I remember all the times my father called my mother stupid. In a letter to me when she was sixty-three she wrote, "It is a bad state of affairs that the supposedly number one person in your father's life is mostly treated as brainless, to an extent that after so many years I feel it is better to clam up and not try anymore. I can no longer take the contradiction and belittling after so many years of it."

I remember seeing my mother write her maiden

name and married name over and over on a sheet of paper, as if she were trying to figure out who she was. What right did she have to complain? No one had forced her to give up her career and follow my father. She had four kids and a nice house. Her husband didn't beat her. But by forty she was depressed and talking about dying. She withdrew to her bedroom, drank too much, became dependent on prescription drugs, overdosed on Valium. My father, meanwhile, prospered in marriage and career and was widely regarded as a hero for staying with a sick, impossible wife.

Was my mother sick? She was certainly seen to be sick. There is no question that she failed to thrive. But in my view, there was nothing wrong with my mother that a good dose of compassion wouldn't have cured. What if the doctors had understood the condition of women's lives? What if they had connected her with other struggling married women, or helped her find the purpose of her life outside the role of family caretaker and adjunct to my father? My mother might have had a chance. Instead, they gave her more Valium. The doctors' interventions dug her deeper into her predicament.

What I Saw Inside the Shelter:
A Pattern of Contempt for Women Emerges

I got the job at the shelter. I don't know what I thought I was getting into, but I was not prepared for the horrors I began to witness on a daily basis. Lucy Stone's "disappointment speech" was made in 1855 at a U.S. women's rights convention in response to the charge that the woman's movement was that of "a few disappointed women." I still love the word disappointment; it captures a kind of pain most women relate to. But soon I had to find new words: words to describe the most appalling violations of women's bodies and souls. I began to witness cruelty so extreme it challenged my belief in what it means to be human. I never got used to it.

Many Canadians think serious violence against women only happens in far-flung places where women have no rights. The reality is that every day in this country, in communities urban, rural, and remote, women are assaulted by men they know and love. They are beaten with authority and entitlement, and seldom with a drop of remorse. Often it is women's request for fair play that triggers a battering incident, though the submissive and self-effacing are beaten too. Women may be assaulted sparingly – a disciplining slap or kick, a gob of spit – or with titanic fury.

I saw women with their faces split open, with broken noses, teeth and jaws, shattered eardrums, bruised necks, sliced and severed fingers. I saw full boot prints on women's thighs, backs, and stomachs. I saw women with head injuries from baseball bats and tire irons, and bowels leaking from penetration with steel rods. Women on my watch were thrown from moving cars, locked outside in sub-zero temperatures, kicked while pregnant, battered while undergoing cancer treatment, choked until blood vessels burst in their eyes. I attended funerals and vigils for women who had been bludgeoned, strangled, scalded, and stabbed to death, shot with gun or crossbow, drowned, suffocated, poisoned, run over, thrown off balconies. Some women were hunted down and slain like animals. Sometimes their murders were made to look like accidents or suicide. Sometimes they were murdered along with their children. Women's bodies were desecrated and disposed of like garbage – rolled up in old carpets, stuffed in hockey bags, strewn in ditches, incinerated in burning cars and houses or in the fire pit in the back garden. One woman's husband cut up her body with a chain saw. The body of a woman in her seventies was found in a septic tank. She left a journal describing her weeks at the shelter as the best time of her life.

I saw all of this, and more. I could go on about the sexual abuse, about women raped after childbirth or while sick, sleeping, or grieving. A woman with a terminal illness was photographed and raped by her husband despite the drainage bag attached to her kidneys. The violence knew no bounds. I could go on, too, about the mental abuse and the constant death threats and the threats to take women's children, and about how men routinely degrade women by calling them cunts, sluts, and whores. Almost every woman I have worked with has been called these names. Women describe the emotional abuse as worse than the physical because the wounds never heal.

In the face of all this contempt and rage aimed at women, those of us who worked to shelter and protect women were constantly accused of hating men. Similarly, the women who were its victims were regularly accused of making up stories because they were "mentally ill." Women living with abuse do become distressed and many do seek professional help, but abusive men use their wives' visits to doctors against them as "proof" that they are mentally unstable. Bogus though these claims are, they may bring women's credibility and capacity to parent into question.

I also witnessed a persistent pattern of indifference to women at all levels of the justice system. The exceptions only proved the rule. Abused women are regularly forced to jump through hoops to get someone to listen. Batterers are sporadically charged, ineffectively restrained, and inadequately sanctioned. Rapists are rarely charged, those charged seldom convicted. On the other hand, women who strike their partner to defend themselves or their children are regularly hauled off to jail as the state applies its mandatory charging policy in a gender-neutral way.[2]

This is just a partial list of harms.

Without the principled support of police and courts, women have little way to escape the tyranny of abusive men. Many don't make it out alive. In Canada, a woman is murdered by her intimate partner every six days, with women most likely to be killed at the point of separation. These killings send a terrifying message to every woman thinking of leaving a controlling man.

But most abused women are not murdered after separation. They are bullied, harassed, and often terrorized. Post-separation tactics include assault on access visits, threats, intimidation, stalking, and surveillance. A woman never knows when her irate ex-partner will come crashing through a patio door, or enter in stealth through a basement window. Batterers regularly use their children as pawns in their struggle for dominance, refusing to pay support, dragging their ex-wives endlessly through court, maliciously reporting them to child welfare services, and so on. Mothers are constantly forced to hand over children to abusive men, with little regard for their or their children's welfare and safety.

For countless women the road out is long and hazardous, knocking many more years off their lives, depleting their financial resources, damaging their health, separating them from – and often destroying – their children. It seems the harder women try to protect their children in family court, the more they are portrayed as bitter and vengeful, and the harder the axe falls.

Indeed, what is women's mental health supposed to look like in this context?

What Else I Saw in the Shelter:
The Power of Women Coming Together

It is profoundly humbling to have to turn for help to strangers because you are under threat from your own husband. No woman wants to be in a shelter. She goes because she is out of options. She needs to end the relationship and fears she cannot do so safely. But there is relief at being safe and believed, and hope found among people who treat you like a person, with feelings and a mind of your own.

We did not regard women as sick or crazy. "You are a sane person responding to a crazy situation," was our motto. Women's experience was received with empathy and compassion. We gave women a lot of time. It takes time to open up after years of being silenced. We learned to deepen the disappointment in women's hearts, validating injustices and traumas long buried. We marvelled at women's resilience. We helped them rediscover their strength and regain confidence in their own decision-making. And we respected their choices. Many women told us they had been to psychiatrists, psychologists, marriage counsellors, had been medicated, hospitalized, etc., but only in the shelter did they find the kind of support that allowed them to take back their lives.

One of the great benefits of the shelter is that it brings women together, out of silence and isolation.

Standing in the kitchen peeling potatoes they begin to talk about what they have been going through at home. Women may not grasp the fact of their subordinate status, but they feel the injustice in their marriages; they feel acrimony and resentment. In the shelter they meet women of different ages, races, religions with similar narratives of abuse. We ran weekly support groups to help women reflect on their experience in a more structured way, using books and films. Before long, women would come to see their problems as common and social as opposed to individual and psychological. That which had lurked just below conscious awareness was becoming visible.

I struggled to answer the many complex questions that arose. Why are women treated so cruelly? Where does all this rage against women come from? Why do so many otherwise decent men seem to lack a moral compass when it comes to women? Why does women's pain seem to count for nothing?[3] Why do many women not realize they are being abused? Why do so many women spend years covering for brutal husbands? Why is the justice system largely deaf to women's cries for mercy?

When I met Helen Levine the answers to these questions started to become clearer. Her work forced me to look deeper into the structures that lay beneath women's lives. She taught me ways of working that overturned most of what I had learned.

Connecting the Personal and Political[4]

I was the supervisor for social work students on field placements at the shelter. Helen was a social work professor and faculty liaison at the Carleton University School of Social Work. We met regularly with students to discuss their learning. The students and I quickly realized that Helen was committed to ways of working that reduced distance between student and teacher, counsellor and client. She eschewed the role of all-knowing expert and sought to demystify the counselling process.

Helen had thought long and hard about women's status in a patriarchal world and drew a link between many of women's so-called "mental health problems" and the subservient roles assigned to them. She saw anger and depression as natural responses to the inequality, injustice, and low expectations built into women's lives. I had never met anyone with such powerful empathy for women. Being in on a discussion with Helen was always electrifying as she shone light into the dark corners of women's lives, making us see glaring truths. As one student put it, "Patriarchy is a strong force, and Helen effortlessly explains the trickle down and the connection between the personal and the political."

Her insights began with her own life. Helen published numerous articles about women and psychiatry, but the one people remember most includes entries from the diary she kept when she was hospitalized for depression in the 1970s. Helen hated the medical model used by the mostly male doctors, with its emphasis on pathology, weakness, and neurosis. Writing helped her survive the hospital experience – she took to it furiously, "unable to stop the flow of words." So did connecting with other female residents, and reading Phyllis Chesler's *Women and Madness*,[5] the groundbreaking work exposing the connection between women's "mental health problems" and their subordinate status in a male-defined and dominated world. Helen carried the book around like a shield. The feminist framework helped her realize that many of the issues she and other female residents were struggling with stemmed from, or were exacerbated by, their auxiliary status as women.

In the 1960s, Phyllis Chesler, an intern in a New York mental hospital, noticed a double standard of mental health and illness for men and women. The qualities of a healthy adult person – independence, self-determination, confidence – were encouraged in men and suppressed in women, while the giving up of self, dependence, and insecurity groomed in women were part of the profile of the unhealthy adult. She saw how psychiatrists frequently privileged the male perspective and encouraged women to adjust to unjust and restrictive roles, and how women who failed to adjust were diagnostically pathologized. She cited examples of "uncommonly stubborn, talented and aggressive" women hospitalized for not following the rules, their religions, or their husbands. Chesler found that most women committed to asylums were not insane but suffocating within the institution of marriage and the family. The book was an indictment of the medical model and existing definitions of insanity.

Helen realized her survival depended on a drastic reordering of the private sphere. The house had come to symbolize women's powerlessness and subservience as wives and mothers. Out of hospital she entered into negotiations with her husband. She would no longer shop, cook, or clean. "I was no longer willing to collude in the oppression of myself or other women," she said. Freed from the demands of the domestic sphere, Helen went on to a full career at the School of Social Work where she fashioned her ideas into a variety of courses. She developed and formalized the feminist approach to counselling,[6] and wrote and spoke widely on women's issues. She was on the founding board of Ottawa's first shelter for battered women. Her work on marriage and motherhood, radical at the time, continues to resonate with women from all cultures and walks of life.

Motherhood was particularly challenging to deconstruct. Being a mother was for Helen, as it is for many women, a rich and joyful part of life. Why then, she asked, do mothers so often become depressed? She struggled to describe the painful splits, contradictions, and assumptions that surround women in the nuclear family. Helen helped me to see that the unpaid work of the family, which includes physical labour and the job of interpersonal relationships, is the only labour assumed to be undertaken for love and by one sex exclusively, without training, fixed hours, sick leave, vacation, or benefits. It is simply assumed that the woman will appropriately yield her name, mobility, paid job, and financial independence to become wife and mother. These conventions are so rooted in our culture that women no longer forced to relinquish their names continue to do so out of love and tradition. Women are conditioned to view marriage and motherhood as the primary task of their lives, gradually coming to view happiness within restrictive and limiting contexts. "Often it is the absence of severe problems with a mate, rather than the presence of a rich and challenging life, that is seen as the good life for women."[7]

The politics of the family, Helen was saying, robs most women of an independent, adult life. It is not just that women are overloaded with the work of the family – most women now doing double-duty. It is that this is all that is expected of them. This is changing slowly in some places, but for the majority of the world's women the bar remains set very low, eroding confidence, stifling imagination, limiting their ability to dream, let alone achieve. Where creativity and potential are stifled, depression emerges. Women are then sent to psychiatrists to help them "adjust." And the cycle continues.

Conclusion:
A Feminist Approach to Working with Women

When we remove the veil that obscures women's subordinate status, we are left with some urgent questions. How are we to think about women's mental health? Is the mentally healthy woman the one who functions well under unjust conditions, or the one who breaks down? Is she the one who resists and rebels, or the one who adjusts and accommodates? If the backdrop against which women are forced to construct their lives is unseen and unnamed, how are women to understand their own feelings and behaviour?

Feminist counselling replaces traditional mental health assumptions with a personal and political understanding of distress. A feminist approach refuses to blame women or to define their personal struggles in terms of individual pathology. Pain and distress are redefined in terms of the society that has shaped them. Individual struggles are explicitly connected to the collective experience of all women. Women's anger and rebellion are harnessed as strengths.

Feminist counselling is rooted in justice for women. Part consciousness-raising, part sociology lesson, the counsellor makes visible the universal conditions of women's lives, helping women see and liberate themselves from the control and limits placed on them. The underlying assumption is that given a critical lens through which to view their experience, women can begin to understand and take back their lives. The central goal is to empower women, helping them become agents of change in their own lives and in society. Women are encouraged to pursue their dreams and fulfill their potential as separate, self-governing human beings.

This paper has focused on several key areas that give rise to distress in women (marriage and motherhood, violence in intimate relationships, and discrimination in justice and mental health systems) simply because these are areas I have studied in depth. The principle elaborated – that of the social and political conditions operating unseen on women's lives – applies equally to every area of life. The links between women's "poor mental health" and their subordination in religion, sport, the workplace, politics, the media, advertising, the beauty and fashion industry, etc. are the same.

A feminist approach can, and should, be adopted into the practice of psychiatrists, psychologists, physicians, social workers, psychotherapists, and counsellors. Working with women's strengths and resilience, appealing to their intellects, helping them know their own history, connecting them to other women, challenging the systems that harm them: this is the prescription for meaningful and lasting change. There is no better medicine we can offer women than to help them understand the condition of their own lives.

(I am indebted to the great feminist activist and thinker Helen Levine for hundreds of conversations about the politics of women's mental health over thirty years of collaboration and friendship, and for teaching me to keep women at the centre of my practice.)

References

1. Mitchell, Juliet. (1971). *Woman's Estate*. Harmondsworth, U.K.: Penguin.

2. In Ontario, the "zero-tolerance" charging policy introduced in 1994 reflected the gendered nature of intimate partner violence and was intended to protect women and children.

3. Germaine Greer calls women's tears "the cheapest fluids on earth."

4. Thanks to Rachel Levine-Katz for her excellent essay on her grandmother's life and work: "Helen Levine and Her Evolution Towards Feminist Counseling," submitted for SOWK 5801, Carleton University, 2013.

5. Chesler, Phyllis. (2005). *Women and Madness* (30th Anniversary Edition). New York: Avon.

6. Levine, Helen. "Feminist Counseling: A Woman-Centered Approach." Women, Work and Wellness, Alcoholism and Drug Addiction Research Foundation, 1989, pp. 227-252.

7. Levine, Helen and Estable, Alma. (1980). *The Power Politics of Motherhood*. Ottawa: Carleton University.

Post-Script

The Language of Laughter

Allison Crawford

In this collection *Much Madness, Divinest Sense,* the second anthology of women's writing edited by Nili Kaplan-Myrth and Lori Hanson, the notion of *Women Who Care* is expanded to include the perspectives of women with experiences of mental illness. Reading through the vastness and infinite forms and richness with which the authors in this book render their experiences, I was reminded of an essay, written forty years ago, "The Laugh of the Medusa," by Hélène Cixous. I first read Cixous' essay in the 1990s at a very foundational point in my own life. In it, Cixous writes, "I shall speak about women's writing: about *what it will do,*" and she exhorts women: *Woman must write her self: must write about women and bring women to writing, from which they have been driven away as violently as from their bodies − for the same reasons, by the same law, with the same fatal goal. Woman must put herself into the text – as into the world and into history – by her own movement.*

Is it not exhilarating and daunting at the same time that women are still taking up this injunction? There is still an absence of women being fully in "the text" of history, and no perspective is less represented than the experiences of women that relate to mental suffering and illness.

Kaplan-Myrth and Hanson take exciting risks in bringing this writing together. Their risks are both in bringing the personal in such close proximity to the professional, but in also navigating perspectives that are "polluted, heart-wrenching, stigmatized, [and] messy." This writing inhabits realms that have historically been relegated to the margins, doubly marginalized in the intersection of gender and madness – realms of the body, of the inchoate, of emotion, of institutions, of enclosure. These are the realms of the medusa: too terrible to look at, outside of language, incomprehensible within reason, feminine. The medusa's laugh is an utterance that also defies the usual order of language.

And yet, all of the writers in this volume do wrestle with language to represent and bring their experiences to light. They write from perspectives of "patients," family members and caregivers, researchers, health care professionals, and also as students of health care who are learning to take on their professional roles. Kaplan-Myrth and Hanson allow these perspectives to come to the reader in a variety of forms, from personal narrative, memoir, essay, and research paper. The editors do not try to constrain the writers' voices or impose their own order on the pieces. The forms and the voices are as multiple as the personal and embodied experience of psychological suffering and illness. Just as there is no one "woman," there is no one experience of mental illness.

As a reader, I experience the body as it leaks onto the page, escaping from the grappling of language. At times this is uncomfortable: accompanying Bea Leaderman as she pees into a box of Kleenex in her therapist's office; Diane Reid's tormented sleepless body that "raged with self-hatred"; Kay Tyler "breaking down"; Kathy Evans' "franticness" and "storms that ravaged"; and the empty, disconnected postpartum body of Kayla Bathgate, among others.

But language, and the power of this book that brings this language to us, allows sharing. Through expressing the self, each writer conveys her experiences in a way the reader can relate to and have empathy for. One of the things that struck me as a reader was not how strange or fantastical these women's experiences are, but how human, how relatable. This is not the realm of "the other," but of the often overlooked every day that could affect any of us. While experience remains unspoken, and thus unwitnessed, it can be maddening and isolating. As Linda E. Clarke so poetically voices, the garments of secrecy are the garments of shame. Through the struggle of relaying their inner life, each of these writers defeats the shame and isolation that have too long accompanied mental illness and suffering.

Most importantly, in silence and secrecy there can be no sharing that leads to empathy and understanding. There can be no authentic meeting of people. No care. The theme of care still configures this anthology. In order to extend care we need to hear from each other, need experience to be made intelligible. And yet, to do so is a risk. This risk is recounted by many writers in this anthology who took risks to communicate their suffering to doctors, their family, and others, and were met with lack of care or empathy, with silencing or revulsion. Kaplan-Myrth and Hanson direct their preface to "you, as a validation of your struggles and experiences." They invite the telling of these life stories, but they pair it with witnessing and validation. The you is also wide enough to encompass us all.

Another experience as a reader emerged through negotiating the confining spaces of mental suffering in many of these narratives. Under the desk in the locked therapist's office in Bea Leaderman's account; wearing the constricting garments of secrecy that Linda E. Clarke narrates; Diane Reid's dark spaces of mania; the isolated cab of the truck in the parking lot with Kay Tyler; the waiting room under the scrutiny of "terrified, staring" eyes that Shannon Evans recounts; the margins of poverty as a single mother; inside the mental health system, in its wards and offices; a retreat to rooms when suffering leads people to withdraw.

Each perspective allows a new vantage point for the reader to critically (re)consider our preconceived and accepted ideas about what mental illness is and its space within our social worlds. Each vantage point is also willingly precarious as these writers struggle with their own understandings, and as personal experience meets the wider world of social norms and roles, and is renegotiated. The authors join this book just as they negotiated the socially confined spaces of mental illness – not content to remain in the dark and silent spaces allotted them. This navigation through mental illness is not just one of personal surfacing, breaking through, or rejoining the social order. Individually and collectively this book creates new space for protest and action. Many of the writers use their writing as a vehicle to question the system in which mental illness is treated. Julie Strong reflects on what it is like to be a provider within a flawed and underresourced system. Madeleine Cole and Yvonne Boyer decry the lack of mental health services that are responsive to Indigenous women's needs, and services that are ignorant of cultural and historical context. Kate Malachite, Mary Anne Bain, and Sana Sheikh question the limitations and abuses of pharmaceutical treatments. Gustafson, Parsons, Meaney, and Winsor use story as research to show how the system, and its lack of care, creates mental suffering. All of these authors reveal not only the humanity of their own care, but also expose the systemic impediments to care.

I return to Cixous' opening words in her own essay: "I shall speak about women's writing: about *what it will do*." This anthology is a collection of women's writing that gives voice to the often isolating, inchoate anguish of the body, mind, and spirit. It is also a call to *do* something different and to have a different relation with caring and with mental illness. This writing collectively demonstrates that it is not simply enough to care; these authors and this book use their care to catalyze change. This anthology creates new space, and a commons of people that includes all of us touched by mental suffering and illness. Although the writing is by women, it is also a space into which men are invited. But this commons is not one governed exclusively by reason, and drugs, and diagnostic manuals. It is a common space in which the body, emotion, and care have a place. And throughout the space I can hear resounding laughter – the language of warmth, authenticity, and connectedness – calling people out from dark places.

References

Cixous, Hélène. (1976). The laugh of the medusa. *Signs*, *1*(4), 875-893.

Contributors

Mary Anne Ruth Bain continues to embrace her life's journey. She prays with clients at a Catholic Healing Clinic. She has given her heart to Matias, a child she sponsors in Chile. She has opened her home to prayer meetings and to visits from the young people who have become family. But Mary Anne most of all has the heart to be present to her sisters and brothers, the marginalized, who frequent the streets and the shelters of her urban neighbourhood.

Kayla Bathgate grew up in a small, rural Alberta town with her parents and two brothers. Immediately following high school, she met the love of her life and they started their beautiful life together. Kayla and her husband are the proud parents of a fur-baby named Chester and a wonderful little boy, William. Kayla enjoys spending her spare time with family and friends and has a huge appreciation for a good afternoon nap.

Yvonne Boyer, J.D. L.L.M., L.L.D.(Ph.D.), is the Canada Research Chair in Aboriginal Health and Wellness and a Professor of Native Studies at Brandon University. She is a member of the Métis Nation of Ontario and owns Boyer Law Office, where she specializes in providing holistic services that blend mainstream law with Indigenous laws. She has a background in nursing and has published extensively on the topics of how Aboriginal and treaty law intersects with the health of First Nations, Métis, and Inuit. She is the mother of four and grandmother of three.

Joanna Brant has been the Executive Director of the Sexual Assault Centre of Brant in Brantford, Ontario, since May 1995.

Carol Casey, R.P.N., B.A. (Gerontology) is currently working on a degree in adult education. She supports her poetry habit by working in a community care agency, where she is lucky enough to be able to provide educational opportunities for personal support workers whom she considers to be some of the unsung heroes/heroines of the health care system. She wrote "The Escape" after crawling away from a dark time in her life. She has been walking and dancing ever since.

Cathrine E. Chambers, B.A., M.Ed., is a Ph.D. candidate at the Institute of Feminist and Gender Studies at the University of Ottaw and is a feminist psychotherapist specializing in violence against women. Her current research explores the intersection of Indigenous and feminist approaches to healing from trauma and seeks to contribute to a growing body of theoretical scholarship in critical trauma studies that challenges the usefulness of hegemonic understandings of trauma, particularly as they relate to racialized and gendered subjects.

Linda E. Clarke has been a writer and performance storyteller for thirty years. She teaches storytelling and her work has been published and broadcast. Most recently, she is working on a play at the Cleveland Clinic based on her story of neurosurgery which she co-authored with Michael Cusimano, her former neurosurgeon.

Madeleine Cole, B.Sc., M.D., CCFP, has worked in Indigenous communities in Canada as a locum and a family doctor, as well as in Sudan for Doctors Without Borders. She now lives and loves and practises medicine in Iqaluit, Nunavut, where she continues to be challenged by northern medicine and by learning Inuktitut. She has a longstanding commitment to sexual health and reproductive rights. She is also the Director of Medical Education for Nunavut and looks forward to the day when she has Inuit physician colleagues working in Nunavut.

Allison Crawford, M.D., FRCPC, is a psychiatrist at the Centre for Addiction and Mental Health and an Assistant Professor at the University of Toronto. She is also a Ph.D. candidate in the Department of English at University of Toronto, and uses the arts within mental health care. She is a co-founder and Editor-in-Chief of *Ars Medica: A Journal of Medicine, the Arts and Humanities* (www.ars-medica.ca).

Kathy Evans is a mental health advocate. She speaks on behalf of the Schizophrenia Society of Saskatchewan to help break down stigma related to schizophrenia and bipolar illness. She is a caregiver for her schizophrenic/bipolar daughter and bipolar mother. She is also administrative staff in the Department of Community Health and Epidemiology at the University of Saskatchewan.

Shannon Evans is a student at the University of Saskatchewan pursuing a Bachelor of Social Work. She speaks as an advocate for the Schizophrenia Society of Saskatoon and hopes to one day work in counselling related to mental health. Shannon also kayaks, cooks, travels, and writes food blogs.

Rebecca Godderis, Ph.D., is an Associate Professor of Community Health and graduate faculty in the Social Justice and Community Engagement Master's program at Wilfrid Laurier University.

Diana L. Gustafson, M.Ed., Ph.D., is a Professor of Social Science and Health in the Faculty of Medicine, and affiliate faculty in the Department of Gender Studies at Memorial University, St. John's, Newfoundland. Together these positions allow her to pursue her commitment to health-related social justice issues in teaching and research, with a particular interest in women's health and well-being. This is her fourth career. In the not-too-distant future, she is planning a fifth life as an amateur golfer and fiction writer. She expects that her partner, children, four amazing grandchildren, and extended family will continue to be her biggest cheerleaders.

Marty Hamer is a daughter, a mother to two wonderful sons, and a retired child-care worker who believes in the accomplishments of children. She has taught the simple joys of knitting, sewing, and singing to the children in her care and in retirement she now spends time working on her "mother stories." Hey, Mom, this one's for you.

Lori Hanson, Ph.D., is Associate Professor in the Department of Community Health and Epidemiology at the University of Saskatchewan and mother of two sets of grown-up twins. Her academic interests and life experience include community activism, gender and development, global health equity, sexual and reproductive health, health promotion, and transformative education. Her doctoral work involved post-modern life history research with women activists. She loves reading stories (especially by women).

Stephanie Irwin, M.A. R.P.T, is a psychotherapist in private practice. She has interest and experience in working with women and their families during the reproductive years. Her two daughters and life partner have inspired her to continue to advocate for a safe world for parents. Her two dogs remind her to laugh every day.

Donna F. Johnson, M.Ps., is a psychologist who has worked with women struggling to make sense of their lives in a variety of contexts including a battered women's shelter, a family counselling agency, and a police crisis unit. She taught Feminist Practice at the Carleton University School of Social Work for many years.

Nili Kaplan-Myrth, M.D., CCFP, Ph.D., is a medical anthropologist and a family physician. She has spent her academic and professional career talking to people about their experiences of health and illness, their bodies, their emotions, and their personal and community well-being. She runs her own busy feminist medical clinic and she retreats to the cottage at the end of each week to play guitar with her husband and curl up for games and stories with their three children.

Esther Kohn-Bentley, M.Ed., is a psychotherapist and coach in Toronto. She is CEO of Panoramic Feedback, a company which provides an online tool for assessing leaders in organizations. Outside of work, she visits with her mother, volunteers as a counsellor for families of people with dementia, and loves to act, sing, sail, and spend time with her husband, children, and grandchildren.

Bea Leaderman is a pseudonym, as the author has been advised to remain anonymous.

Kate Malachite is a pseudonym, as the author prefers to remain anonymous.

Patricia Meaney has worked in the hospitality industry, as a research assistant, and as a full-time solo parent to her two sons. She is currently taking a break from her post-secondary studies but upon return plans to pursue a career in social work. A passionate and engaged community activist, Patricia has contributed to varied public education and advocacy initiatives with lone mothers and anti-poverty activists as well as charitable community events and political campaigns. In her spare time, she enjoys motorcycle riding around Newfoundland, and the company of friends.

Sheila C. Morrison, B.A., B.Sc. (Physiotherapy), M.A. (Health Education), retired teacher and physiotherapist, spent many years as an advocate for change in the mental health care system. She is currently caregiver for her adult daughter and a writer of essays and short fiction. She enjoys acting and singing and, along with her husband, daughter, and her daughter's service dog, exploring Nova Scotia's beaches and woods.

Janice E. Parsons, M.S.W., R.S.W., is an Assistant Professor in the School of Social Work, and Faculty Associate with the Centre for Collaborative Health Professional Education at Memorial University. Her commitment to working collaboratively with lone mothers and allies toward the eradication of poverty and stigma is nurtured by her practice and research experience with lone mothers, and her personal experience of having been raised by an inspiring lone mother. Sailing, gardening, and learning about science and dinosaurs with her four grandsons are some of her favourite activities.

Diane Reid, B.A., currently lives on disability but worked for many years as a fiddle teacher as well as for non-profit organizations. She has been living with mental illness for fifteen years and is grateful for the people who have stayed with her through her ups and downs. She treasures spending time with her happy, healthy adult son.

Kylie Riou, M.D., is a psychiatry resident at the University of Saskatchewan. She is passionate about mental health awareness and reducing stigma in her career and everyday life. In her own wellness journey she practises yoga, meditation, and meaningful time with family and friends.

Sana Sheikh, Ph.D., completed her graduate studies in social psychology at the University of Massachusetts Amherst and is pursuing her license to practise clinical psychology. Her scholarly interests span psychological perspectives on emotion and morality with a focus on the social and cultural nature of emotional experience and its implications for psychiatric nosology and treatment.

Julie Strong, M.D., CCFP, is a family physician in Halifax, Nova Scotia. She is also trained as a shamanic practitioner. Strong's queer tragicomedy, *Athena in Love*, earned Best Playwright's Award in the Atlantic Fringe Festival, 2012, and she won the short story award in the Atlantic Writing Competion in 2010. An excerpt from her memoir features in *Letting Go, an Anthology of Attempts*, Bacon Press, Washington D.C., 2016. She loves drumming and creating transformative space.

Kay Tyler is a small-business owner and has an unquenchable curiosity about the world around her. She and her wife live in a little house with a big garden and their lives are filled with music, friends, and family.

Jayne Melville Whyte, B.A., is a mental health educator and advocate. Jayne wrote *Pivot Points: A Fragmented History of Mental Health in Saskatchewan* with the Canadian Mental Health Association (CMHA Saskatchewan, 2012) and continues researching the contribution of consumer/survivors in mental health movements. Participants in her workshops explore new paths for communication and action among psychiatric survivors, service providers, and policy-makers. Jayne resides in the beautiful valley of Fort Qu'Appelle.

Cherish Winsor, a corporate communications specialist, divides her time amongst a wide range of community and social policy projects. Her work tends to focus on issues related to low-income populations, women and children, and homelessness. Her political aspirations help to keep her an informed and engaged community member. Along with her husband and five children, Cherish is enjoying the adventure of life near the beautiful Arctic tundra in Canada's Northwest Territories.